How to see Your Health

NOTE

This book about the oriental art of visual diagnosis is part of a series introducing the infinite order of nature that eternally governs all phenomena and all lives throughout the universe.

It follows *The Book of Macrobiotics: The Universal Way of Health and Happiness*, published in 1977, which presents the understanding and applications in the biological realm of the principles of the order of the universe, especially the development of health and happiness.

The Book of Dō-In: Exercise for Physical and Spiritual Development, published in 1978, introduces physical and spiritual exercises for self-development according to the same principles.

Natural Healing through Macrobiotics, published later in 1978, explains the causes and methods of treatment of various physical and mental disorders. Also published in 1979, *How to Cook with Miso* by Aveline Tomoko Kushi presents ways of cooking healthful foods following these natural principles.

Following the above publications, this book, *How to See Your Health: The Book of Oriental Diagnosis*, reveals methods for seeing everyone's health through visual observation. After this substantially useful book, another volume—*Oriental Psycho-diagnosis for Health and Happiness*—will be presented. This forthcoming book will elucidate human emotional and psychological life and the understanding of the energy, vibrations and waves which compose and decompose our daily life in the form of psychological phenomena.

How to See Your Health:
Book of Oriental Diagnosis

MICHIO KUSHI

Japan Publications, Inc.

© 1980 in Japan by Michio Kushi

Published by JAPAN PUBLICATIONS, INC., Tokyo

Distributors:
UNITED STATES: *Kodansha International/USA, Ltd., through Harper & Row, Publishers, Inc., 10 East 53rd Street, New York, 10022.* SOUTH AMERICA: *Harper & Row, Publishers, Inc., International Department.* CANADA: *Fitzhenry & Whiteside Ltd., 150 Lesmill Road, Don Mills, Ontario M3B 2T6.* MEXICO AND CENTRAL AMERICA: *HARLA S.A. de C. V., Apartado 30–546, Mexico 4, D. F.* BRITISH ISLES: *International Book Distributors Ltd., 66 Wood Lane End, Hemel Hempstead, Herts HPZ 4RG.* EUROPEAN CONTINENT: *Boxer books, Inc., Limmatstrasse 111, 8031 Zurich.* AUSTRALIA AND NEW ZEALAND: *Book Wise (Australia) Pty Ltd., 104–8 Sussex Street, Sydney 2000.* THE FAR EAST AND JAPAN: *Japan Publications Trading Co., Ltd., 1–2–1, Sarugaku-cho, Chiyoda-ku, Tokyo 101.*

First edition: November 1980
Second printing: May 1981

LCCC No. 79–89346
ISBN 0–87040–467–9

Printed in U.S.A.

Preface

Knowing is the beginning of freedom.
The art of knowing is the art of
  realizing freedom.
All suffering comes from ignorance:
Ignorance of what I am, ignornace of
  who I am, of what we are.
The art of knowing is the opening
  of the secret of life,
And a path for health, happiness and
  eternal life.

December 25, 1979

This book is intended for all people, non-professionals as well as professionals in the medical, psychological and physiotherapeutic sciences. My purpose in writing this book is to present the basic principles and arts of diagnosis, which can be practiced without using any of the measures harmful to physical and mental well-being that are applied frequently in the modern medical sciences.

From time to time throughout the book, the phrase "oriental diagnosis" is used, referring to the fact that the principles underlying these arts were developed and preserved in Japan, Korea, China and India among religious, cultural and philosophical traditions for many centuries. They can be found in *The Book of Changes* (易経, *I Ching*), *The Yellow Emperor's Classic of Internal Medicine* (内経, *Nei Ching*), *The Tao Teh Ching* (道徳経), the *Karaka Samhita*, the *Kojiki* (古事記), the *Nihon-Shoki* (日本書紀), and numerous other classics in these countries, and as a cosmological source of Hinduism, Buddhism, Zoroastrianism, Judaism, Confucianism, Taoism, and Shintō. These principles are the Law of the Universe, or we can say *the order of the infinite universe*, which operates perpetually throughout the dimensions of this universe: producing, changing, decomposing, and demolishing all phenomena, including phenomena from this earth.

When the order of the universe was applied to the metaphysical phenomena of humankind, it developed the various religions. When it was applied to natural phenomena, it developed the sciences. Applied to human relations, it developed moral codes, ethics, and economics. When it was applied to human esthetic manifestations, it developed the cultures and arts; and when it was applied to the problems of health, it developed the various domains of the medical arts, including the art of diagnosis.

However, these applications—which as a whole created the way of life of the ancient peoples of the world, and the way of life in the Orient until a few centuries ago—have decayed and disappeared, due to the newly arisen modern ways of thought and technology, which are based mainly upon analytical, divisional and materialistic views, and which have rapidly spread and prevailed since the sixteenth century during the westernization of the world.

After experiencing the modern scienctific, technological and materialistic civilization, it has become clear that the very existence of life on this planet may be endangered by the rapid degeneration of human health in the modern world, and that the life sciences, including the modern medical approach, have been inadequate to preserve human well-being from such universal decline. Not only internal treatments and external surgical applications, but also the techniques of modern diagnosis itself, are frequently harmful to human health. In view of these circumstances, the renaissance of traditional wisdom based upon a more total comprehension of cosmology, including the arts of health and diagnosis, has become absolutely essential to recover humanity, individually and collectively.

When it became clear to me as a student of world peace, pursued through research in political science, that the reconstruction of humanity is the decisive factor in laying the foundations for the development of a unified world, I began to study the natural order of humanity, encouraged by several senior teachers— namely Mr. George Ohsawa, the Rev. Dr. Toyohiko Kagawa, Prof. Shigeru Nanba, and others—and discouraged by the lack in modern educational facilities of teachings on the medicine for humanity. I began to stand on the streets in New York City—on 42nd Street and Broadway around Times Square, and on 5th Avenue—observing thousands of people: their body structure, their way of walking, their way of expression, their faces, their behavior and their thinking. In cafeterias and restaurants, theaters and amusement parks, trains and subways, shops and schools, every day I observed the countless variety of human manifestations on this present earth. Week by week, month by month, and year by year as time passed, it became very apparent that all physical, psychological, social and cultural manifestations of human activities depend upon our environment and dietary habits. It became clear that even so-called hereditary factors are nothing but the result of the past environment within which our ancestors lived, and what they were observing as their daily diet.

I noticed that in terms of the environment, I had to include not only the immediate natural and social conditions such as the weather, climate, season, city or country, but also a much wider sphere of influence—to the infinite dimensions of the entire universe, in both time and space—in order to understand the human species. I also noticed that in terms of food, I had to include not only the daily material food and drink consumed through the mouth, but also the entire world of inorganic substances, organic biological life, the atmosphere, electro-magnetic forces, and all sorts of waves and radiations coming from all directions from the unknown depths of the universe. The understanding of these factors in relation to our daily condition, I noticed, was only possible by comprehending the order of the universe and its applications, and not by analytical and divisional methods of research.

Since that time, more than twenty-five years have passed, during which I have met hundreds of thousands of people through educational activities, lectures, seminars and consultations on the way of life to recover health and realize total well-being. Encountering these people has revealed a deeper under- standing of human nature, and further understanding of the art of diagnosis has continuously developed this art itself. The information presented in this book is only an introduction of several major methods of diagnosis that anyone can use. Some of them are based upon classical methods, and others are newly developed and interpreted through my personal experience. In writing this book, I have avoided as much as possible the use of technical terminology, for the convenience of many readers. It is my sincere wish that this introductory book may contribute for every reader to understand the present conditions of health of himself, his family, relations, friends and whomever he may en- counter, and may serve as a starting point for society to recover total health and achieve freedom and happiness, toward the eventual realization of one peaceful world.

This book was dictated from June 1979 to January 1980, in Brookline, Massachusetts, with frequent interruptions for European and American lecture tours, seminars, classes, personal counselling and many other activities to promote the evolutional development of modern people through the under- standing of the order of the universe, and the use of natural healthful food oriented with macrobiotic principles—the equivalent of the order of the uni- verse. The assistant who typed, edited and corrected the original English ver- sion of the book is Miss Olivia Oredson of Brookline, Massachusetts, who is currently the educational director of the Kushi Institute. The Kushi Institute is an educational organization for the study of the order of the universe and its applications for the development of humanity, through the establishment of health by various natural ways of healing, with the comprehension of the nature of humanity and the total destiny of mankind in all major domains. Illustrations and drawings in this book were composed by Mr. Joe di Gregorio of Brookline, Massachusetts; Miss Lily Kushi of Brookline, Massachusetts; and the author.

> When everyone reads everyone else,
> Love and compassion prevail.
> When everyone reads the art of nature,
> Health and peace prevail.
> Unwritten words are living everywhere,
> And they are coming forth from the
>   universe.
> When we read them all without missing
>   a single word,
> We have opened the book of the sevcret
>   of eternal life.
>   MICHIO KUSHI
>   December 26, 1979

Order in Making Diagnosis

Step 1: DESTINY.   Whether a person is happy or not, and whether he or she will become happy or not.

Step 2: PERSONALITY. What kind of ideals, view of life, nature and character he or she has.

Step 3: CONSTITUTION.   What kind of constitution he or she has, both physically and mentally.

Step 4: DISORDERS.   What kinds of disorders he or she has developed and suffers at present.

Step 5: RECOMMENDATIONS.   What changes are required to turn his or her disorders into health and well-being.

Step 6: ORIENTATION.   To what kind of future should he or she be oriented to realize happiness.

Step 7: INSPIRATION.   What encouragement should be given to develop his or her endless possibility to achieve happiness.

Contents

Part One

The Principles of Diagnosis

1. The Order of the Universe

From ocean to continent,
From desert to mountain,
From flower to animal,
From space to time,
Everything is governed
By the Universal Law.
Yin and yang are everywhere;
Without them, nothing exists
And nothing changes.

December 26, 1979

All phenomena in this universe and upon this planet earth are manifestations of the infinite law of the universe, which is the law of change, the law of manifestation. Because of these laws, everything in the world manifests out of the infinite ocean of non-existence, and demanifests into this ocean again. The laws of the universe, in a simplified modern version, can be represented by seven theorems of the absolute world, and twelve principles of the relative world, although they are all manifestations of one infinity:

The Seven Universal Theorems
1. Everything is a differentiation of one Infinity.
2. Everything changes.
3. All antagonisms are complementary.
4. There is nothing identical.
5. What has a front has a back.
6. The bigger the front, the bigger the back.
7. What has a beginning has an end.

The Twelve Principles of Relativity
1. One Infinity manifests itself into complementary and antagonistic tendencies, yin and yang, in its endless change.
2. Yin and yang are manifested continuously from the eternal movement of one infinite universe.
3. Yin represents centrifugality. Yang represents centripetality. Yin and Yang together produce energy and all phenomena.
4. Yin attracts yang. Yang attracts yin.
5. Yin repels yin. Yang repels yang.
6. Yin and yang combined in varying proportions produce different phenomena. The attraction and repulsion among phenomena is proportional to the difference of the yin and yang forces.

7. All phenomena are ephemeral, constantly changing their constitution of yin and yang forces; yin changes into yang, yang changes into yin.
8. Nothing is solely yin or solely yang. Everything is composed of both tendencies in varying degrees.
9. There is nothing neuter. Either yin or yang is in excess in every occurrence.
10. Large yin attracts small yin. Large yang attracts small yang.
11. Extreme yin produces yang, and extreme yang produces yin.
12. All physical manifestations are yang at the center, and yin at the surface.

In order to understand the relative laws of the relative world, the following classifications of the antagonistic and complemental tendencies, yin and yang, show practical examples of these relative forces operating in the relative world.

Examples of Yin and Yang

	YIN ▽*	YANG △*
Attribute	Centrifugal Force	Centripetal Force
Tendency	Expansion	Contraction
Function	Diffusion	Fusion
	Dispersion	Assimilation
	Separation	Gathering
	Decomposition	Organization
Movement	More inactive, slower	More active, faster
Vibration	Shorter wave and higher frequency	Longer wave and lower frequency
Direction	Ascent and vertical	Descent and horizontal
Position	More outward and peripheral	More inward and central
Weight	Lighter	Heavier
Temperature	Colder	Hotter
Light	Darker	Brighter
Humidity	More wet	More dry
Density	Thinner	Thicker
Size	Larger	Smaller
Shape	More expansive and fragile	More contractive and harder
Form	Longer	Shorter
Texture	Softer	Harder
Atomic particle	Electron	Proton
Elements	N, O, P, Ca, etc.	H, C, Na, As, Mg, etc.
Environment	Vibration ... Air ... Water ... Earth	
Climatic effects	Tropical climate	Colder climate
Dimension	Space	Time

* For convenience, the symbols ▽ for Yin, and △ for Yang are used.

Attribute	YIN ▽ Centrifugal Force	YANG △ Centripetal Force
Biological	More vegetable quality	More animal quality
Sex	Female	Male
Organ structure	More hollow and expansive	More compacted and condensed
Nerves	More peripheral, orthosympathetic	More central, parasympathetic
Attitude, emotion	More gentle, negative, defensive	More active, positive, aggressive
Work	More psychological and mental	More physical and social
Consciousness	More universal	More specific
Mental function	Dealing more with the future	Dealing more with the past
Culture	More spiritually oriented	More materially oriented
Dimension	Space	Time

The classification shown above of the different forces and tendencies is only one example of similar classifications of phenomena. Universal relativity, namely yin and yang, is relative in its very nature, and there can be no absolute classification and definition of yin and yang—antagonistic and complementary factors—in any one chart, because of the dynamic nature of change and the complex constituents of every substance. Many other classifications of relative forces can be produced: for example, based upon activity and movement, or based upon vibrational and energetic character, or based upon physical and material nature.

Application of the Order of the Universe

The order of the universe and its principles described above can be directly applied to the art of diagnosis, because human beings are one of the biological and spiritual manifestations on this planet in this infinite universe. The application of these theorems and principles in the art of diagnosis can be summarized in the explanation that follows:

1. *All physical, mental and spiritual manifestations of human beings are manifestations of the environment.*

Changes in the environment, including changes in cosmic rays, radiations, waves and vibrations received from celestial movements and the infinite depths of the universe, and changes in the more immediate physical environment such as atmospheric conditions, weather, climate, seasons, months, and hours, all influence the changes in our physical and mental conditions.

2. *The part of the environment taken into the body composes the internal environment, in balance with the external environment.*

All factors assimilated into our body from the environment—electromagnetic energies, vibrations, air, water, minerals, as well as plant and animal life—compose our internal condition, forming our skeletal, muscular and organ constitutions by the generation of trillions of cells, through our digestive and circulatory functions in coordination with our respiratory, excretory and nervous activities.

3. *The balance between the external environment and the internal environment creates physical and mental states.*

Between the external environment which expands to the infinite dimensions of space and time, and the internal environment which is organically compacted and created from substances of the external environment, there is constant inter-action. In the event such interactivity becomes either abnormally over-active or underactive, it produces disorders in the physical and mental conditions and activities. When outgoing energy is more active than incoming energy, it manifests as growth and maturity as well as expanding and overactive conditions of various organs; while if outgoing energy becomes less than incoming energy, it manifests as aging and contracting underactive conditions of organs.

4. *Physical manifestations can be classified as constitutions and conditions.*

The factors received from the parents and ancestors in the form of reproductive cells, and the development during the pregnant and growing periods—which is primarily a repetition of the entire process of biological evolution from a single cell to a complex human being—form the constitution, that is, our fundamental character and tendencies. The factors we consume every day, especially during the recent period of about seven years, and more so within the past three to four months, including daily consumption of food and drink, compose our condition. Although all factors of our constitutions and conditions are changeable, constitutions change far more slowly, while conditions change rapidly with daily physical and mental variations.

5. *There are numerous antagonistic and complemental relationships within our physical and mental constitutions and conditions.*

Because everything is composed of antagonistic and complemental factors and tendencies, yin and yang, and everything operates due to the change of relationships between these opposing factors and tendencies, human physical and mental manifestations are also constituted and function by these two opposing factors and tendencies. Examples are listed in the following chart:

STRUCTURES

More Yin ($\triangledown$)	*More Yang* ($\triangle$)
Part of body	Part of head
Front of body or head	Back of body or head
Soft parts	Hard parts
Expanded organs	Compacted organs
Peripheral parts	Inner parts
Upper position	Lower position

FUNCTIONS

Nervous functions in general	Digestive functions in general
Electromagentic meridian functions	Fluid circulation functions
Sympathetic nervous functions	Parasympathetic nervous functions
Female functions	Male functions
Mental activities	Physical activities
Eliminating functions	Consuming functions
Ascending movement	Descending movement
Differentiating, outgoing movement	Gathering, incoming movement
Expanding movement	Contracting movement
Exhaling function	Inhaling function
Flexible movement	Inflexible movement
Slower movement	Rapid movement

These parts of the body and functions are balancing each other in their structural formation and operational functions, according to the aforementioned twelve principles of relativity.

6. *Foods and drinks forming the internal environment can be classified on a scale according to their antagonistic and complemental relationships.*

Foods and drinks, in their capacity of bringing about the antagonistic and complemental functions listed in the table above, stimulating certain parts of the body and inducing certain functions, can be generally classified as in the table on the next page:

7. *A yin quality of food and drink produces yin structures and functions, while a yang quality of food and drink produces yang structures and functions.*

According to the quality of food and drink in our daily diet, our condition changes daily in proportion. Food and drink cause changes in blood quality and nervous reactions, resulting in changes in structure in the long run, and changes in functions over a shorter period. Simple examples include the expansion of blood capillaries and active elimination of sweat and urination (yin function) as a result of over-consumption of liquid (yin), and the constriction of tissues, nerves and vessels (yang function) caused by overconsumption of salt (yang). There are numerous variations in the reactions, effects, and degree of influence, either yin or yang, of the kinds, combinations and methods of cooking of foods and drinks. Physical and mental activities are also factors that accelerate a more yang condition, while resting and sleeping, especially together with overconsumption of foods and drinks, result in the creation of a more yin condition.

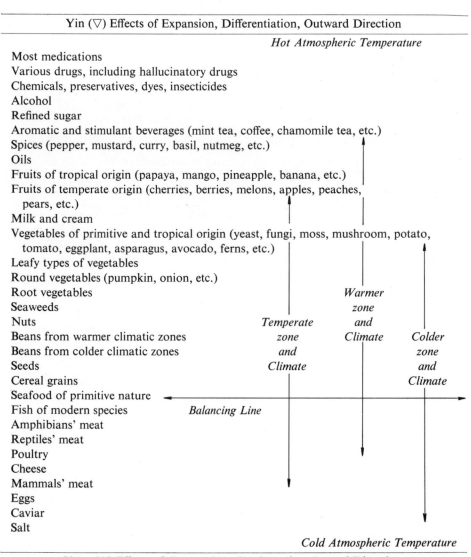

Yin (▽) Effects of Expansion, Differentiation, Outward Direction

Hot Atmospheric Temperature

Most medications
Various drugs, including hallucinatory drugs
Chemicals, preservatives, dyes, insecticides
Alcohol
Refined sugar
Aromatic and stimulant beverages (mint tea, coffee, chamomile tea, etc.)
Spices (pepper, mustard, curry, basil, nutmeg, etc.)
Oils
Fruits of tropical origin (papaya, mango, pineapple, banana, etc.)
Fruits of temperate origin (cherries, berries, melons, apples, peaches, pears, etc.)
Milk and cream
Vegetables of primitive and tropical origin (yeast, fungi, moss, mushroom, potato, tomato, eggplant, asparagus, avocado, ferns, etc.)
Leafy types of vegetables
Round vegetables (pumpkin, onion, etc.)
Root vegetables
Seaweeds
Nuts
Beans from warmer climatic zones
Beans from colder climatic zones
Seeds
Cereal grains
Seafood of primitive nature
Fish of modern species
Amphibians' meat
Reptiles' meat
Poultry
Cheese
Mammals' meat
Eggs
Caviar
Salt

Warmer zone and Climate

Temperate zone and Climate

Colder zone and Climate

Balancing Line

Cold Atmospheric Temperature

Yang (△) Effects of Contraction, Condensation, Inward Direction

8. *The Principle of the Five Stages of Transmutation of Energy.*

In the phenomenal world, energy transforms its manifestations into various forms, including all relative phenomena. All of these phenomena manifested as transitory appearances of energy can be classified into five general states of transformation, between expansion (yin) and contraction (yang).

These five stages are (1) upward expanding motion; (2) very expanded and active motion; (3) condensation process; (4) solidified state; and (5) melting and floating stage (Fig. 1). These stages can be interpreted using characteristic examples seen in daily life:

	Energy	*Examples*
1.	Upward expanding motion	Gaseous state—Tree
2.	Very expanded, active motion	Plasmic state—Fire
3.	Condensation process	Semi-condensed state—Soil
4.	Solidified state	Solid state—Metal
5.	Melting and floating state	Liquid state—Water

Fig. 1   Five Stages of Energy Transformation

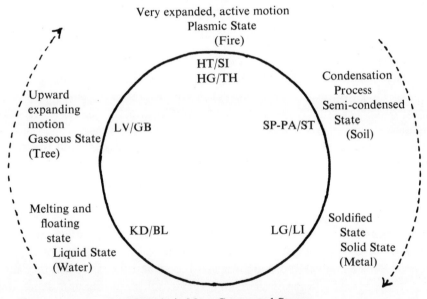

Yin (▽), Most Expanded Stage

Yang (△), Most Contracted Stage

LV/GB—Liver and Gallbladder
HT/SI—Heart and Small Intestine
HG/TH—Heart Governor and Triple
Heater functions (Circulatory and Heat Metabolism)

SP-PA/ST—Spleen, Pancreas and Stomach
LG/LI—Lungs and Large Intestines
KD/BL—Kidneys and Bladder

These five stages of changing energy also reflect the energy functions related to various organs and meridians, as illustrated in Fig. 2.

Fig. 2 Five Progressive Activations of Energy According to Season and Time of Day

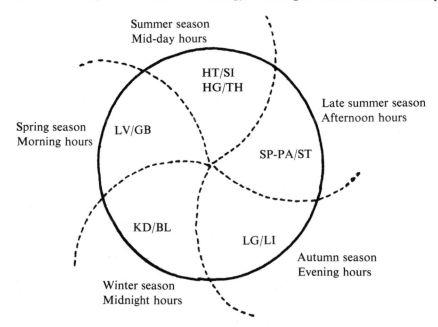

These energy conditions are also related to seasonal energy change, monthly or lunar energy change, and daily energy change, as well as environmental conditions. They also describe psychological conditions, and dietary effects. The chart of energy conditions on opposite page is directly related to the study of diagnosis.

The foods listed in this chart nourish and activate the organs and functions of the same category. For example, wheat, barley, young leafy vegetables and sprouts can nourish and accelerate the functions of the liver and gallbladder. Also, physical disorders appear more obviously as symptoms in the features belonging to the same category. For example, disorders of the lungs and large intestine appear more clearly in the nose and skin conditions as well as in the breath. They also create a pale facial color, a fishy odor, and other physical phenomena such as snivel and coughing. At the same time, they produce more changes in the voice; and psychologically, they result in crying and depression with a feeling of sadness.

Furthermore, using this table, we can easily diagnose physical conditions. For example, if the head hair is in an abnormal condition (bushy or fragile, etc.), or if there are aches and pains in the bones, or disorders in the ears or the hearing, major disorders are indicated in the kidneys and bladder, or in the excretory functions.

The Five Transformations of Energy

	A	B	C	D	E
Energy:	Upward	Very active	Downward	Solidified	Floating
Examples:	Gas	Plasma	Condensation	Solid	Liquid
	Tree	Fire	Soil	Metal	Water
Organ Energy:	Liver, gall-bladder	Heart, small intestine	Spleen-pancreas, stomach	Lungs, large intestine	kidneys, bladder
Direction:	East	South	Center	West	North
Season:	Spring	Summer	Late summer	Autumn	Winter
Time of month:	Increasing half-moon	Full moon	Obscured moon	Decreasing half-moon	New moon
Time of day:	Morning	Noon	Afternoon	Evening	Night
Environment:	Windy	Hot	Humid	Dry	Cold
Grain:	Wheat, barley	Corn	Millet	Rice	Beans
Vegetables:	Sprouts and upward-growing plants	Enlarged leafy plants	Round plants	Contracted, small plants	Root plants
Fruits:	Spring fruits	Summer fruits	Late summer fruits	Autumn fruits	Winter and dried fruits
Odor:	Oily, greasy	Burning	Fragrant	Fishy	Putrefying
Tastes:	Sour	Bitter	Sweet	Pungent	Salty
Physical parts:	Tissues	Blood vessels	Muscles	Skin	Bones
Physical branches:	Nails	Body hair and facial color	Breast, lips	Breath	Head hair
Skin color:	Blue, grey	Red	Yellow, milky	Pale	Black, dark
Physical liquids:	Tears	Sweat	Slaver	Snivel	Saliva
Physical changes:	Gripping	Anxious	Sobbing	Coughing	Shivering
5 Voices:	Shouting	Talking	Singing	Crying	Groaning
5 Functions:	Color	Odor	Taste	Voice	Fluid
Psychological reaction:	Anger, excitement	Laughing, talkative	Indecisive, suspicious	Sadness, depression	Fear, insecurity

This table also shows changes in the environment by the season, month, day and atmospheric conditions. Accordingly, diagnosis can be made. If a fever arises regularly at a certain hour, or on a certain day of the month, or in a certain season, it indicates that the organs listed in the same energy category are the primary location of the disorder. For example, if a sickness occurs in a very humid atmosphere, especially on the afternoon of a cloudy day, it indicates that the spleen and stomach are involved as the major problem organs.

In order to alleviate these physical and mental disorders, we can emphasize a change in diet toward the foods belonging to the same category, and an avoidance of the foods listed in the opposite categories. For example, in the case of diabetes, which involves the functions of the pancreas, an increase in foods such as millet and round vegetables—cabbage, pumpkin, hard squash, and others—would be recommended as an important part of the dietary approach.

2. Constitution and Condition

The Constitution and Its Order

The human physical and mental constitution is formed with the following influences:

—hereditary factors from the reproductive cells of the mother and father.
—mental and physical influences from the mother during pregnancy.
—nourishment through food and the environment during growth after delivery.

In connection with these factors forming the constitution, the following influences must be well considered for the purpose of diagnosis to understand anyone's condition and destiny:

A.   Parental and ancestral conditions.
B.   The quality of the reproductive cells.
C.   The date of conception and birth.
D.   The place of birth and growing.
E.   The food that the mother ate during pregnancy, and the food eaten during the growing period.
F.   Family, social and cultural influences.

Let us examine these factors in detail.

A. Parental and ancestral conditions.   In the event the physical and mental conditions of the ancestors and parents are more physically oriented, including their daily work and way of life, their offspring would have similar tendencies, unless there has been a major change in diet, residence, and social and cultural influence before or during the period of pregnancy. On the other hand, more mentally and spiritually oriented ancestors and parents tend to produce offspring more characterized by similar mental and spiritual tendencies. These similar characteristics are especially evident if the family has maintained similar traditions and living situations under similar climatic conditions with similar dietary practices through the generations.

B. The quality of the reproductive cells. The reproductive cells—the sperm and egg, especially their quality before fertilization—are a fundamental factor for the development of the future physical and mental constitution. Not only DNA, RNA and other genetic factors, but also the quality of the vibrations, energy, nutritional makeup and other constituent factors of the reproductive cells serve as the beginning of human development. In connection with this influence, the following principles apply:

1. *The sex of the child.* In the event the sperm are more active than the egg, a female child will be more likely; while if the egg is more energized, a male child will be the result.

2. *Major systems in the child's body.* Because the father's sperm tends to contribute a stronger influence to the child's nervous system, while the mother's egg gives more influence to the digestive and reproductive systems, the constitution of the newborn child will vary in its coordination among the nervous, digestive and reproductive functions according to the differences in quality in both reproductive cells.

3. *Major organs in the child's body.* The father's influence through his sperm tends to appear more on the left side of the child's face and body, including the left lung, left atrium of the heart, spleen, pancreas, stomach, left kidney, left side of the small intestine, descending colon, and left ovary or testicle. The mother's influence through her egg tends to manifest more in the right side of the head and body, including the right lung, right atrium of the heart, liver, gallbladder, right kidney, the duodenum, right side of small intestine, ascending colon, and the right ovary or testicle.

4. *The child's mental and physical nature.* The father's influence appears more in the child's intellectual, social and ideological character, while the mother's influence appears more in the child's physical, sensory and emotional character, during and after the growing period as a whole.

C. The date of conception and birth. The date of conception and birth have a very important influence upon the formation of the physical and mental constitution. This has been studied in the traditional arts of oriental and western astrology as one of the ways of seeing destiny. In practical terms, seasonal atmospheric conditions including the electromagnetic charge on the ground, in the water and air, as well as radiations, waves and other vibrations coming from celestial movements, give different influences to the quality of the parents' physical and psychological conditions, and influence their reproductive vitality and the quality of their sperm and egg. In addition, their dietary pattern changes according to the season and month, oriented by the movement of the earth, sun, moon and other planets, resulting in different qualities of the blood cells that produce the reproductive cells.

These dietary changes continue during pregnancy as the seasons progress, either from hot to cold or cold to hot. This climatic change has a strong influence on the mother's dietary pattern during the nine-month period. Therefore, a child born in the spring will have a physical and mental constitution that is opposite to that of a child born in the autumn (Fig. 3).

Fig. 3   Birthdate and Biological Constitution

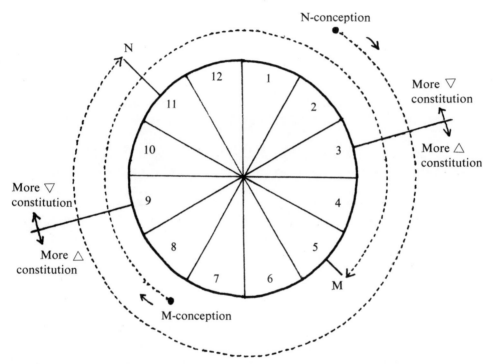

Numbers 1 to 12 indicate the months January through December. M–person, born in the middle of May, began his embryonic period in early August, while N-person, born in November, began his embryonic period in early February.

1.   A person born in May passed his embryonic period from August of the previous year through the winter and spring seasons. During this time, his mother was eating a diet suitable for the fall and winter seasons, including more salty, cooked food and less perishable food, with more animal food in most cases. On the other hand, a person born in November has eaten, through his mother's diet during pregnancy, more spring and summer types of food, including less salt and less cooking, most probably with more fruits, juices, sweets and liquid. These two persons therefore have different biological histories. During the nine months of pregnancy, their constitutions have

developed while they increased nearly three billion times in weight, repeating the entire precess of biological evolution from a single cell to the emergence of life from the water. Their differences are complemental and antagonistic.

2.   Accordingly, any person has a constitution that is antagonistic and complemental to that of a person born in the opposite season and month. These differences can serve as supportive tendencies, although these two persons may often have difficulties in understanding each other. Persons born in the same month or same season share similar physical and mental constitutions and tendencies. They can understand each other more easily, although their attraction may be less than that of people born in very different months and seasons.

3.   It is not surprising that people born in the same or similar month or season share the same or similar physical and mental disorders, more so than people born in very different months or seasons:

—Among those born in the spring and summer, there is a greater potential to develop bronchitis, lung tuberculosis, and other respiratory disorders; kidney and excretory disorders; and heart and circulatory disorders.

—Among these born in the autumn and winter, there is a tendency to develop digestive disorders, especially in the liver, gallbladder, spleen, pancreas and small intestine; sicknesses such as diabetes, constipation, diarrhea, stomach and duodenal ulcers, and other sicknesses related to these organs; and nervous disorders.

These differences in data of conception and birth can be categorized into two large, general groups: spring- and summer-born nature, and autumn- and winter-born nature. The dividing line falls in early March and early September.

D.   The place of birth and growing.   The place of birth and growing is important to consider in diagnosing general physical and mental tendencies. Environmental and atmospheric conditions strongly influence the dietary practices during the period of pregnancy and growth after birth, resulting in significant dietary differences among those who are born and grow in a warmer climate and those who are born and grow in a colder climate. The former tend to eat more light, less-cooked foods including raw vegetables, fruits and juices, and sweets, while the latter tend to eat more salty, well-cooked grains, beans and vegetables with more animal food.

Such differences can also be observed among people who originate near the seashore, those who come from the plains, and those who come from the mountains. Those who were born and grow near the sea tend to eat more seafood; those from the mountains tend to eat more well-cooked food; and people from the plains tend to eat a more average diet.

We can also see important differences between city-born and country-born people. Those who were born and grow in the city, especially in modern times, have consumed more mass-produced, commercial foods; while those who were born and grow in the country ate foods of more natural quality.

From these differences related to the place of birth and growth, different physical and mental constitutions develop which show tendencies for certain disorders:

Place of Birth and Growth	*Potential Disorders*
More northern, colder region; more mountainous area	Skin diseases; accumulation of mucus and fat; formation of tumors and growths; disorders in the liver and gallbladder.
More southern, warmer region; areas near the sea	Disorders in the intestines, lungs, kidneys and bladder, as well as reproductive and nervous sicknesses. Some skin diseases and tumors. Paralysis and arthritis.
City areas	Complex disorders, especially in the intestines, lungs, and nervous functions, as well as in the reproductive organs.
Country areas	More simple and distinct disorders. Fewer digestive, reproductive and nervous disorders.

E. Diet during pregnancy and growth. The quality of the food consumed during the periods of pregnancy and growth has a decisive effect upon the formation of the constitution, determining all features of body forms and structures, character and personality, the capacity and functioning ability of the organs and glands. General tendencies are as follows:

Kinds of Food Eaten	*Tendencies*
Grains, beans and cooked vegetables	Generally harmonious metabolism, physically and mentally active and balanced. Fewer disorders. More intuitive and esthetic nature.
Vegetables, especially less-cooked or raw	More gentle and skeptical. Disorders in skin conditions, respiratory and excretory functions; chronic intestinal disorders.

Kinds of Food Eaten	*Tendencies*
Fruits, juices and nuts	More sentimentality, nervousness, sensitivity; critical nature. Disorders and tendency to weakness in the intestines and digestive functions and reproductive organs.
Dairy food	More gentle, slow mind; dull response. Skin disease, formation of mucus, fat; heart and circulatory disorders; liver, gallbladder and spleen disorders; reproductive disorders; more cysts, tumors and cancer formation.
Meat, poultry and eggs	More stubbornness and exclusivity, determination; more material interest. Sharp senses. More mechanical abilities. Heart and circulatory disorders, small intestine and digestive disorders, formation of tumors and cancer.
Sugar, honey and other sweets	Mental illusions, schizophrenia, nervousness, obesity, diabetes, skin disease, various disorders in the sensory organs and nervous system, chronic digestive disorders, kidney and excretory disorders, reproductive weakness.
Spices and stimulants	Irritability, emotional insecurity, abnormal blood pressure, heart and circulatory disorders, kidney and excretory disorders, some skin diseases, irregularity in reproductive functions.

F. *Family, social and cultural influences.* In the formation of the physical and mental constitution, the traditional way of living practiced in the family, immediate community, and general culture, along with the influence of education, has an important influence. These factors regulate the way of eating in a certain traditional pattern, as well as the way of behavior and thinking.

For example, immigrants to North America have a tendency to maintain the traditional ways of eating and behavior practiced in their original countries, during the first and second generations in America. Also, religions such as Catholocism, Protestantism, Buddhism, Islam, Judaism, Hinduism, Taoism, and Confucianism have a traditional influence on dietary, moral and ethical behavior. Buddhist followers tend to eat more grains and vegetables, while Protestants have a variety of dietary practices. Judaism includes a practice of customary dietary habits, and followers of Islam tend to use more oily and spicy foods.

Education can also contribute to the change of dietary and social habits. While those who receive less education tend to follow more traditional family practices, those who follow more education tend to liberalize their dietary and social behavior, including a wider variety of nutritional supplements, with commercial foods. In this regard, the level of prosperity of the country or society also contributes to the population's change of dietary and social behavior. As a result, people's physical and mental constitutions rapidly change as modern educational, cultural and economic conditions change. Those who live in areas isolated from modern development tend to maintain traditional physical and mental constitutions, on the other hand.

2. *Diagnosis of Constitutional Types*

In the art of diagnosis, the constitution can be assessed using several methods. Let's examine some of these methods:

A. Bone structure. The quality of the constitution can be seen more in the bone structure, while the quality of the condition appears more in the muscles, skin, and other peripheral areas of the body. The constitution can be judged by feeling the bones, especially in the area of the shoulders, arms and legs. Stronger and bolder bones indicate a more yang, strong constitution, while thinner and weaker bones indicate a more yin, weak and fragile constitution. The former type of person has a tendency to be more active in physical and social life, while the latter tends to be more active in mental and artistic life.

B. Muscle and skin conditions. Softer muscles show a more yin constitution, nourished by more fluid, vegetables and fruits; while tighter muscles show a more yang constitution, nourished by more grains, beans, and animal food, with more minerals. The condition of the skin is also an indication. However, in comparison with the bones, the condition of the muscles and skin are more changeable through diet and exercise, since they are composed of more protein and fat while the bones are composed of more minerals. Accordingly, while the muscles and skin show the constitution developed during the periods of pregnancy and growth, they also show the present physical and mental conditions. Softer muscles and fine skin indicate a more adaptable and mentally-oriented nature, while tighter and harder muscles and skin show a nature that is more physically oriented and active.

C. The ratio of head to body. The standard proportion of head to body in vertical length is 1:7 (Fig. 4). If the head is smaller, say in a ratio of 1:8, the physical and mental constitution is weaker than average, due to the quality of food consumed during the mother's pregnancy. On the other hand, if the head is vertically larger than average, say in a ratio of 1:6, it shows that the physical and mental constitution is much stronger than average, and there is a tendency to be much more active in both mental and social life.

Fig. 4 Proportion between Head and Body

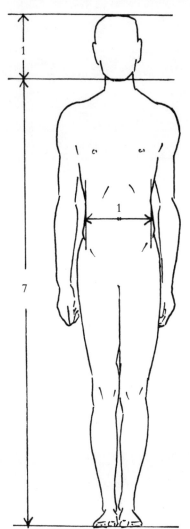

Fig. 5 Height Differences

A—More yang (△) constitution
B—More yin (▽) constitution

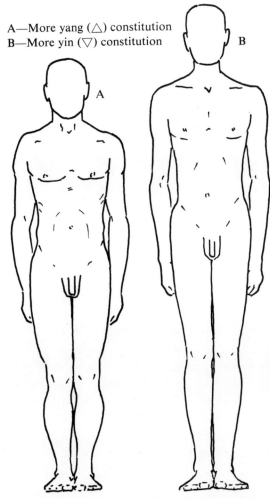

D. Height. Taller people have a more yin constitution, while shorter people have a more yang constitution (Fig. 5). The former tend to develop more mental abilities, and become susceptible to respiratory and nervous disorders. The latter tend to engage themselves in a more active physical and social life, with a tendency to be more susceptible to digestive and circulatory disorders.

E. Angle of the shoulders. Those who have more sloping shoulders have a more feminine character, with a nature of esthetic and artistic appreciation; while those who have more square shoulders have a more masculine character, and tend to appreciate more physical and social activities and more intellectual thinking (Fig. 6). If the shoulders form a more round shape with balanced muscles, it shows a more balanced character embracing both mental and physical activities as well as esthetic and intellectual tendencies.

Fig. 6 Angle of the Shoulders

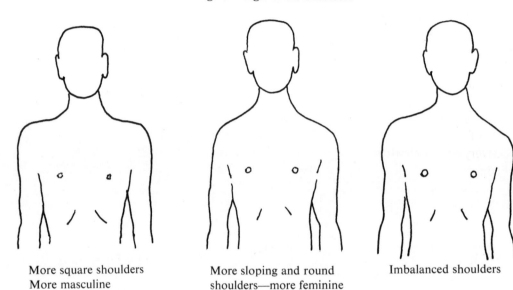

More square shoulders
More masculine

More sloping and round
shoulders—more feminine

Imbalanced shoulders

If the shoulders are imbalanced—one side higher than the other—it indicates that the organs on the side of the higher shoulder are weaker than the organs on the side of the lower shoulder, and especially in the case of the lungs and large intestines.

F. The hands and feet. Larger and thicker hands and feet result from a more yang diet during the time of pregnancy, which produced a strong inner constitution, combined with a more yin diet during the growing period, which produced peripheral expansion. This type of person tends to be strong in the inner physical and mental conditions, but also flexible and artistic in the social and intellectual activity. On the other hand, people with smaller hands and feet show physical strength but less activity in mental life.

Long, sensitive finger and toes show a nature more appreciative of the emotional, artistic and esthetic worlds, while short, stocky fingers and toes show a more physically active nature, with stronger resistance to the environment, but less appreciation for mental and spiritual matters.

G. Other features. Many other physical features can be used to diagnose the constitution, and many of them are discussed later in this book. Among them are diagnosis of the shape of the face and head, the teeth, the size and shape of the mouth and eyes, the length and angle of the eyebrows, the posture and behavior, and other factors.

Antagonistic and Complemental Relations in Human Structure and Function

In diagnosis, practical observations are made by finding the antagonistic and complemental relations in structure and function that appear in the constitution and condition. Among numerous antagonistic and complemental relations, some of the most important are discussed in the following section.

1. The head and face manifest the internal conditions of the body.

A. Face–organ correlations. During the fetal and embryonic period, the navel functioned as the center of the entire body structure. At the time of delivery and thereafter, this center shifted to the mouth and neck region. From this point, upper and lower extensions have developed—the head as the

Fig. 7 Face–Organ Correlations

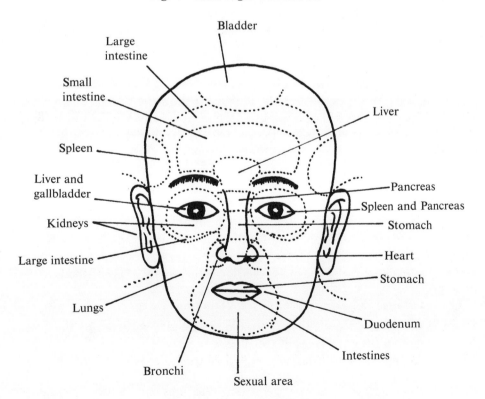

upper sphere and the body as the lower sphere. Accordingly, they correlate with each other very well, the lower part of the head region representing the upper part of the body region (with the exception of the mouth and mouth cavity, which shows the digestive conditions); the middle part of the head region representing the middle part of the body region, and the upper part of the head region representing the lower part of the body. According to this principle, each area of the face manifests each organ and its functions of the body (Fig. 7).

1. The condition of the cheeks shows the condition of the lungs and their functions.
2. The tip of the nose represents the heart and its functions, while the nostrils represent the bronchi connecting the lungs.
3. The middle part of the nose represents the stomach, and the upper part of the nose represents the condition of the pancreas.
4. The eyes represent the kidneys as well as the condition of the ovaries in the case of woman, and the testicles in the case of man. Also, the left eye represents the condition of the spleen and pancreas, while the right eye represents the liver and gallbladder.
5. The area between the eyebrows shows the condition of the liver, and the temples on both sides show the condition of the spleen.
6. The forehead as a whole represents the small intestines, and the peripheral region of the forehead represents the large intestines.
7. The upper part of the forehead shows the condition of the bladder.
8. The ears represent the kidneys: the left ear the left kidney, and the right ear the right kidney.
9. The mouth as a whole shows the condition of the entire digestive vessel. More specifically, the upper lips show the stomach; the lower lips show the small intestines at the inner part of the lip and the large intestines at the more peripheral part of the lip. The corners of the lips show the condition of the duodenum.
10. The area around the mouth represents the sexual organs and their functions.

B. Face–major systems correlations. During the embryonic period, all major systems of the body, namely (1) the digestive and respiratory systems, (2) the nervous system, and (3) the circulatory and excretory systems, gather and form the entire facial structure, sharing four general areas of the face (Fig. 8).

a. The lower part of the face around the mouth, bordered by the lines coming from the sides of the nose.
b. The upper part of the face, including the nose, bordered by the eyebrows.

Fig. 8 Face–Major Systems Correlations

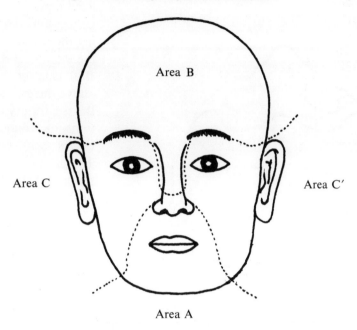

c. and c′.   Both sides of the face, including both eyes, cheeks and ears.

The areas outlined in the illustration above correspond to certain organs and functions in the body, as follows:

Area A: The conditions of the mouth, lips, tongue, mouth cavity, and area around the mouth, show the digestive functions as a whole. This area also relates partially to the respiratory function, especially at its peripheral area.

Area B: The condition of the forehead and its periphery, including the temples and eyebrows, represent the conditions of the nervous system as a whole.

Areas C and C′:   The side facial areas, including both eyes, cheeks and ears, represent the conditions and functions of the circulatory and excretory systems as a whole.

C.   Correlations between the head, systems and organs.   The head region can be divided into several areas, each of which reflects the conditions of certain systems and organs (Fig. 9).

A.   The central part of the head where the hair spiral is located represents the condition of the heart and small intestine.

B.   The area surrounding area A represents the digestive systems and functions, including the esophagus, stomach, duodenum, and large intestines.

Fig. 9   Correlations between Head, Systems and Organs

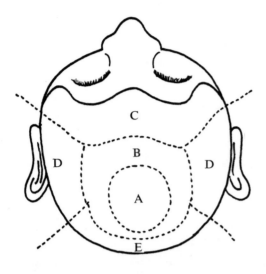

C. The front part of the head represents the excretory functions, including the conditions of the kidneys and bladder.

D. Both sides of the head above the ears show the respiratory conditions, including the lungs and bronchi conditions.

E. The back of the head represents the condition of the liver, spleen, and pancreas.

F. The entire peripheral area of the head represents the circulatory system and its conditions.

D.   Head–buttock correlation.   In connection with the relationship between the upper and lower parts of the body, the head region corresponds to the buttock region for the reason that the head is the upper end of the nervous system and the buttocks are its lower end. Therefore, certain areas of the buttocks correspond to certain areas of the head and brain (Fig. 10). Tension and other abnormal conditions of the brain also appear in the conditions of the muscles and tissues in the area of the buttocks.

Fig. 10   Head–Buttock Correlations

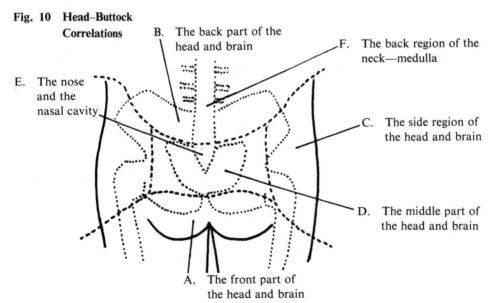

B. The back part of the head and brain

F. The back region of the neck—medulla

E. The nose and the nasal cavity

C. The side region of the head and brain

D. The middle part of the head and brain

A. The front part of the head and brain

   A. The lower buttock region corresponds to the front part of the head and brain.

   B. The upper part of the buttock region corresponds to the back area of the head and brain.

   C. The side buttock regions correspond to the side regions of the head and brain.

   D. The central buttock region corresponds to the middle part of the head and brain.

   E. The coccyx area represents the nose and nasal cavity.

   F. The lower spine near the waist corresponds to the medulla at the back region of the neck.

2. *The peripheral parts of the body such as the hands and feet reflect the condition of the inside of the body.*

   A. The palms. The palms represent the condition of the internal systems and functions as a whole, namely (1) the digestive and respiratory system, (2) the nervous system, and (3) the circulatory and excretory systems (see Fig. 11).

Fig. 11   Palm–Major Systems Correlations

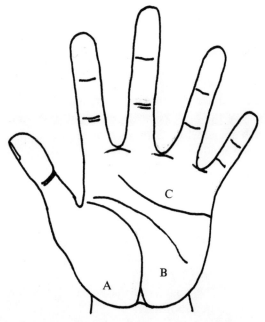

Line A and its related area on the palm at the root of the thumb represents the digestive and respiratory functions, including the condition of the esophagus, stomach, small intestine, large intestine, and lungs.

Line B and the area connected to that line represent the nervous system, including the functions of the brain and central nervous system, and the peripheral nerves.

Line C and its surrounding area represents the circulatory and excretory systems, including the condition of the heart, kidneys and bladder.

Fig. 12   Correlation between the Fingers and Major Systems and Organs of the Body

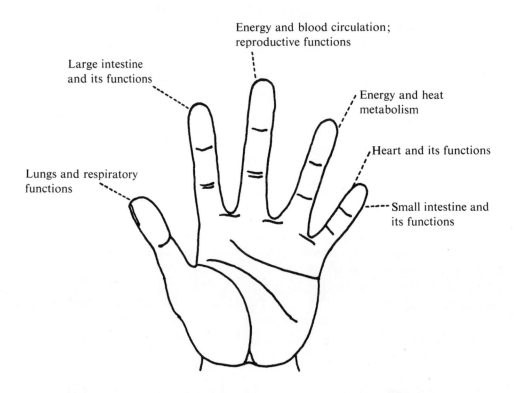

B.   The fingers.   The fingers represent the organs and functions located in the upper part of the body, namely the lungs and heart; and in the lower part of the body, namely the small intestines and large intestines, as well as their related functions such as circulation and heat metabolism. Each finger corresponds to a certain function (Fig. 12).

> The *thumbs* represents the conditions and functions of the lungs and respiratory activities.
> The *index fingers* represent the large intestines and their functions.
> The *middle fingers* represent the energy vitalized around the heart and circulatory functions, including reproductive vitality.
> The *ring fingers* represent the activity of eliminating excessive energy from the regions of the heart, stomach and intestines—energy and heat metabolism.
> The *little fingers* represent the conditions and functions of the heart and small intestines.

C.   The feet.   The feet also represent the condition of the whole body. Since the body and the feet are involved in the body's balance of vertical and horizontal relationships, each part of the feet correlates to each part of the body, and conditions appearing in each part of the feet correspond to the conditions in the organs and functions of the related parts of the body (Fig. 13).

1. Points A, B and C correlate respectively to the kidneys, the heart and stomach, and the abdominal center.
2. The inside ball of the foot (D) under the big toe corresponds to the shoulders and shoulder blades, while the outside ball (E) corresponds to the lungs and respiratory functions.
3. The inside middle region of the foot represents (F) the nose and mouth cavity, (G) the throat and vocal cords, and (H) the bronchi and diaphragm region.
4. The outer middle region of the foot (I) represents the stomach, duodenum, and upper intestinal region.
5. The inner lower region (J) corresponds to the intestinal region, especially the middle part of the intestines.
6. The heel (K) as a whole corresponds to the lower intestinal region, the rectum, and the uterus.
7. The line running along the bottom outside of the foot (L) represents the spine and the muscles along the spine, as well as the meridian related to the bladder functions.

Fig. 13   Foot–Body Correlations

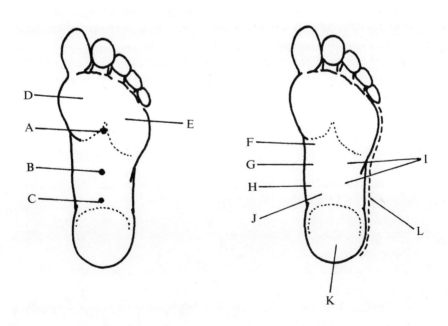

Fig. 14   Toes–Organs Correlations

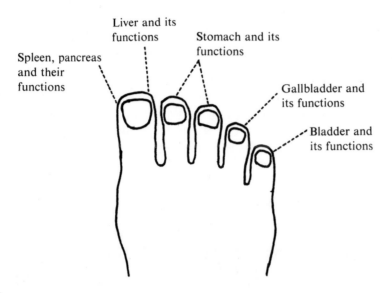

Liver and its functions

Stomach and its functions

Spleen, pancreas and their functions

Gallbladder and its functions

Bladder and its functions

D.   The toes and toenails.   The toes and toenails represent the organs and their functions which are located in the middle region of the body, namely the spleen and pancreas, liver, stomach, gallbladder, and bladder (Fig. 14).

> *The first toe* and its nail correspond to the spleen, pancreas, and their functions, especially the outer area. They also correspond to the liver and its functions, especially at the inner area.
>
> *The second and third toes* and their nails represent the stomach and its functions. The second toe represents more the stomach organ and its functions, and the third toe represents more the functions of the stomach sphincter and duodenum.
>
> *The fourth toe* and its nail correspond to the gallbadder and its functions.
>
> *The fifth toe* and its nail correspond to the bladder and its functions.

On the bottom of the foot, the areas just at the base of each toe correspond to certain organs and functions (Fig. 15).

> *A.*   The area under the second toe: functions of the heart and circulation.
>
> *B.*   The area under the third toe: functions of the spleen and lymph circulation.
>
> *C.*   The area under the fourth toe: functions of the lungs and respiration.

Fig. 15 Areas at the Base of the Toes Correlating with Major Body Functions

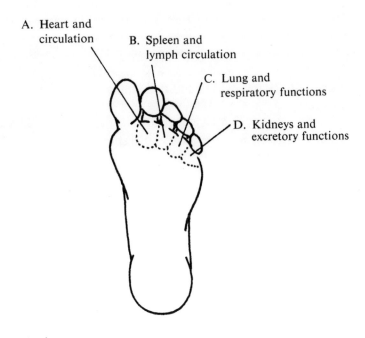

A. Heart and
   circulation

B. Spleen and
   lymph circulation

C. Lung and
   respiratory functions

D. Kidneys and
   excretory functions

D.   The area under the fifth toe: functions of the kidneys and excretory
system.

3.   Conditions in the Front and Back of the Body.

The front and back of the body maintain an antagonistic and complemental
relationship, and each area of the front correlates to each area of the back.
Conditions appearing in the frontal organs reflect conditions in the back, and
vice versa. The following show examples for the purpose of diagnosis.

A.   YU-Entering Points and BO-Gathering Points.   Points located in the
front of the body and points located in the back in connection with certain
organs and functions are known as the *YU*-Entering Points and the *BO*-
Gathering Points (Fig. 16).

1.   These points on the back are known as *YU*-Entering Points, into
     which environmental energy or electromagnetic force spirals, forming
     and feeding energy to the organs and activating their functions.

2.   These points located in front are known as *BO*-Gathering Points,
     which gather the energies that have nourished and functioned in the
     respective organs. Energy gathers at these points, and from them is
     further distributed and eliminated toward the peripheral environ-

ment through the arms and fingers, legs and toes, forming the electromagnetic lines known as *meridians*. These meridians and their electromagnetic flow are used in the various treatments of oriental medicine, such as acupuncture, moxibustion, shiatsu massage, and palm healing.

B. *Correlation between front and back areas.* General areas on the back correlate to certain frontal organs and their functions (Fig. 17).

1. The back of the head (A) correlates to the functions of the eyes and visual processes, and the nose and respiration.

Fig. 16 YU-Entering Points and BO-Gathering Points

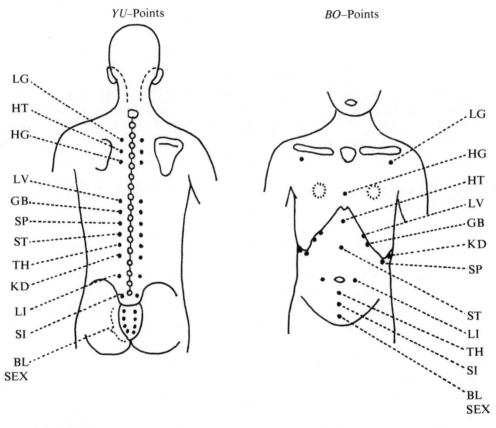

YU–Points

BO–Points

LG—Lungs
HT—Heart
HG—Heart Governor (Energy
    Circulation)
LV—Liver
GB—Gallbladder
SP—Spleen and Pancreas
ST—Stomach

TH—Triple Heater (Energy and Heart
    (Metabolism)
KD—Kidneys
LI—Large Intestine
SI—Small Intestine
BL-SEX—Bladder and
    Sexual functions

2. The back of the neck (B) including the region of the medulla oblongata down to the bottom of the shoulder blades correlates to the mouth cavity, vocal cords and respiratory functions.

3. The upper back (C) thoracic region correlates to the lungs, bronchi and respiratory functions, and the large intestine and its functions.

Fig. 17 Front and Back Correlations

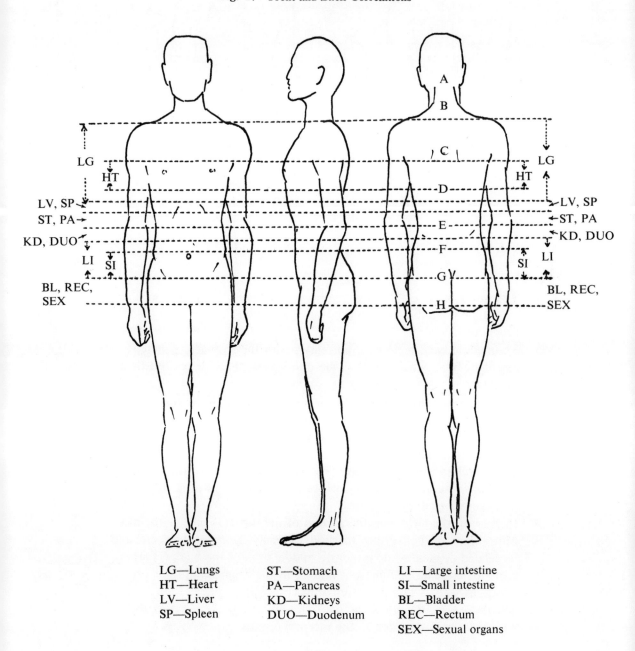

LG—Lungs	ST—Stomach	LI—Large intestine
HT—Heart	PA—Pancreas	SI—Small intestine
LV—Liver	KD—Kidneys	BL—Bladder
SP—Spleen	DUO—Duodenum	REC—Rectum
		SEX—Sexual organs

Fig. 18   Vertical Correlations between Front and Back

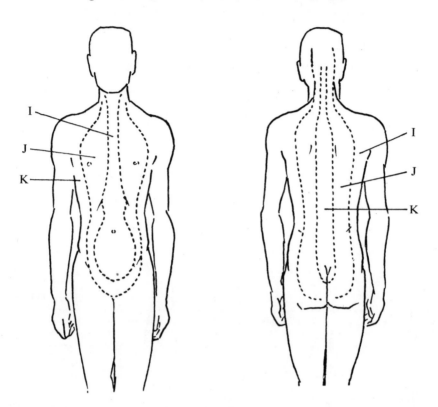

4. The lower back (D) thoracic region correlates to the lower lungs and their functions, the diaphragm, liver, gallbladder, spleen and their functions.

5. The middle back region (E) correlates with the stomach, pancreas and their functions, as well as the duodenum, the kidneys and their functions.

6. The region directly above the waist (F) correlates to the transverse colon, the upper small intestines, and their functions.

7. The waist region (G) correlates to the lower small intestine, ascending colon, descending colon, and their functions.

8. The sacral and buttock region (H) correlates to the rectum and its functions, the uterus, ovaries, prostate, testicles, and other reproductive conditions and functions.

9. In general, the more peripheral area of the back (I) reflects the more central part of the front of the body, namely the digestive vessel and its related organs, while the more middle area of the back (J) represents the circulatory functions related to the organs and their processes, as well as excretory functions (Fig. 18).

10. The more central part of the back (K) represents the nervous system and its functions related to the internal organs.

4. A part manifests the whole.

As the entire human body is a miniature of the universe, a part of the body also is a miniature of the whole body, having the apparent reflection of the conditions of the whole. Practically speaking, from the condition of each organ, it is possible to see the whole body condition. Even a single cell or a single hair represents the condition of the entire body. For diagnostic purposes, it is convenient to know a few examples as introduced below.

A. The eyes. The eyes reflect the condition of the whole body's organs and functions. There is a study called "iridology" which examines the relation between the conditions of the iris and the conditions of the organs. However, it may be more convenient to examine the white of the eye as well, in order to diagnose the whole body's condition. Guidelines are illustrated in Fig. 19.

The outer area of the white, covering sections 1–6, represents the front of the body:

Area 1. The area from the front of the head toward the face.
Area 2. From the face and neck toward the lungs.
Area 3. From the lungs and heart to the stomach, pancreas, liver and spleen.
Area 4. The region from these organs in the middle part of the body to the duodenum and upper part of the small and large intestines.

Fig. 19   Correlations between the Eyeball and Body Organs and Systems

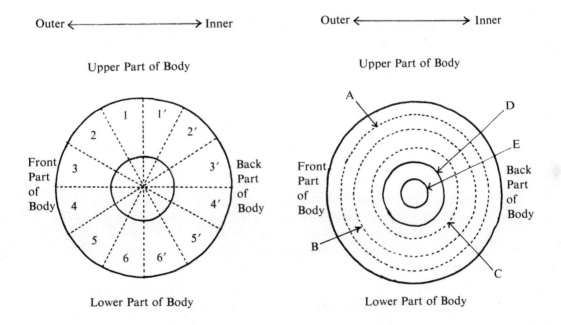

Area 5. The lower part of the intestines.

Area 6. The region of the bladder and reproductive organs.

The inner area of the white covering sections 1'–6' represents the back of the head, neck and body:

Area 1'. The region of the back of the head and brain.

Area 2'. The region from the medulla oblongata to the shoulders and upper part of the back area of the lungs.

Area 3'. From the middle and lower part of the lungs to the liver, spleen and kidneys.

Area 4'. From the kidneys and urethra to the back region of the upper intestines.

Area 5'. The lower part of the intestines, especially the back area.

Area 6'. The bladder and reproductive organs, especially their back areas.

Furthermore, the major systems and their functions appear as follows (refer to Fig. 19):

1. The area along Line A, the outer edge of the white, represents the digestive system and its functions.

2. The area along Line B, the inner side of the white, represents the nervous system and its functions.

3. The area along Line C represents the circulatory and excretory functions.

4. The area along Line D, the outer edge of the iris, represents the autonomic nervous functions, especially of the orthosympathetic nervous activity.

5. The area along Line E, the outer edge of the pupil, also represents the autonomic nervous functions, especially of the parasympathetic nerves.

B. The ears. The ears also represent the whole body and certain parts of the ear manifest the condition of certain organs and their conditions (Fig. 20).

1. Area 1, the upper part of the ear represents the lower part of the body, including the small and large intestines, the bladder, reproductive organs and their functions.

2. Area 2 represents the middle part of the body, including the stomach, liver, spleen, pancreas, duodenum and their functions.

3. Area 3 represents the upper part of the body, including the lungs, heart, bronchi, and shoulders, and their functions.

Fig. 20 Ear–Body Correlations

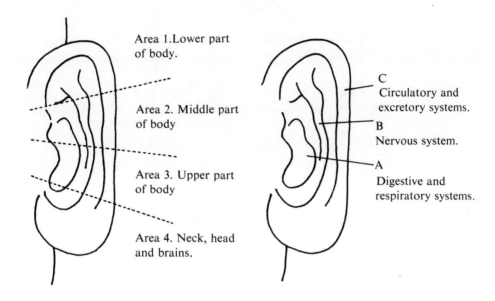

Area 1.Lower part of body.

Area 2. Middle part of body

Area 3. Upper part of body

Area 4. Neck, head and brains.

C
Circulatory and excretory systems.

B
Nervous system.

A
Digestive and respiratory systems.

4. Area 4 represents the head and brain region, including the medulla oblongata, the neck and face and its various organs such as the eyes, nose, ears, mouth, and brain, and the glands in the head region as a whole.
5. The innermost vertical area of the ear (A) represents the digestive and respiratory systems and their functions.
6. Vertical area (B) of the whole ear represents the nervous system and its functions.
7. The most peripheral wing area of the entire ear (C) represents the circulatory and excretory systems and their functions.

C. *The abdominal region.*   The abdominal region can be used for diagnosis by pressure, to detect hardness, tightness, rigidity and pain. Each region of the abdominal area represents the condition and functions of certain corresponding organs (Fig. 21).

Area A: The upper abdominal region represents the conditions of the heart and small intestines.
Area B: The right side of the abdominal region represents the condition of the lungs and large intestines.
Area C: The left side of the abdominal region represents the condition of the liver and gallbladder.
Area D: The lower abdominal region represents the condition of the kidneys and bladder.

Fig. 21   The Abdominal Region and Correlation with Organs

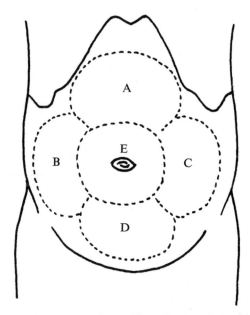

Area E: The central part of the abdominal region represents the conditions of the spleen, pancreas and stomach.

D.   Other organs and features for diagnosis.   Besides the examples outlined above, there are numerous other ways that the condition of the entire body manifests into a certain organ or part of the body. Some of these are:

1.   The eyebrows represent the digestive and nervous systems, and their quality is an indication of longevity.
2.   The lines coming from the sides of the nose and running down toward the mouth manifest the conditions of the digestive and circulatory functions, and are another indicator of longevity and vitality.
3.   The hands and feet each represent the whole body.
4.   The fingerails and toenails represent the functions of the circulatory and excretory systems.
5.   The hair represents the digestive, circulatory and nervous functions.
6.   The teeth correspond to the spinal cord and vertebrae, as well as the organs connected to each vertebra.
7.   The tongue represents the entire digestive, circulatory and nervous functions.

In the following Part 2, we will study these interrelationships in connection with the diagnosis of specific conditions of our physical and mental well-being.

Part Two

Visual Diagnosis of Specific Conditions

A part manifests the whole;
The whole reflects a part.
The small represents the large;
The large corresponds to the small.
Sometimes they appear the same,
Sometimes they appear opposite;
But all of them seem a chorus
To praise the glory
Of the endless universe.

January 6, 1980

The general principles of diagnosis outlined in the previous part 1 lead us to observe and discover the various manifestations of physical and mental conditions. These manifestations show the condition of the internal organs and their functions. The arts of diagnosis outlined in the following section can be used to reflect upon our own condition, and to see the conditions of other people.

1. The Mouth and the Teeth

The Mouth and Lips

The mouth and lips show both the general constitution and the current condition of any person, and especially of the digestive organs and functions. Because the mouth and lips are the beginning of the digestive tract and the entrance for the foods and drinks we consume, they reflect very clearly the internal condition of the digestive tract, as well as the condition of the anus —the end of the digestive tract and the exit for the elimination of any undigested and unabsorbed foods and fluids.

A person who has good physical and mental health and strength will have a mouth that is the same width or narrower than the width of the nose (Fig. 22). This kind of small mouth was predominant among people until a few generations ago, but the mouths of modern people are rapidly becoming much larger, indicating general degeneration of the physical and mental constitution. If a person's mouth is much wider than the width of the nostrils, it shows that the functions of the organs and glands are weak, and both physical and mental abilities for adapting to and resisting the environment are also weak.

The increase in mouth size among modern people is due to the overconsumption of potatoes and tomatoes, fruits and juices, sugar and other sweetners, oil and fat, coffee and other beverages, which were eaten by the mother

Fig. 22 Size of the Mouth

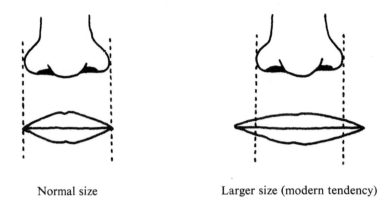

Normal size   Larger size (modern tendency)

and received through the mother's blood during pregnancy. These foods and drinks cause a deficiency of minerals. Over-intake of protein in proportion to the intake of carbohydrate also causes the development of a larger mouth.

The different areas of the mouth and lips correspond to certain areas of the body, and the digestive system in particular (Fig. 23).

—*The upper lip* shows the condition of the upper part of the digestive tract, especially the stomach. The inner part of the upper lip corresponds to both upper and lower ends of the stomach. The peripheral areas of the upper lip correspond to the middle region of the stomach.
—*The lower lip* shows the condition of the lower digestive tract, especially

Fig. 23 Areas of the Lips Corresponding to Certain Organs

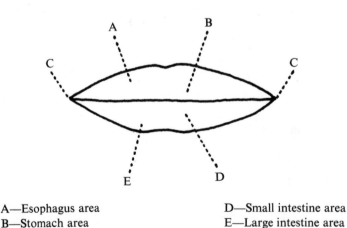

A—Esophagus area   D—Small intestine area
B—Stomach area   E—Large intestine area
C—Duodenum area

the small and large intestines. The inner area of the lower lip corresponds to the condition of the small intestine, and the peripheral areas of the lower lip correspond to the large intestine.

—*The corners of the lips* show the middle region of the digestive tract, especially the duodenum. The right corner corresponds more to the duodenum's reaction to bile secretion from the liver and gallbladder. The left corner reflects more the functions resulting from pancreatic secretions.

1. General Conditions

The size of the mouth, including its horizontal breadth and vertical fullness, shows the general quality of the physical constitution and condition, and especially that of the digestive system (Fig. 24).

Fig. 24   Forms of the Mouth: Width

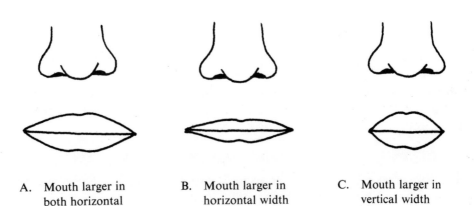

A. Mouth larger in both horizontal and vertical width.

B. Mouth larger in horizontal width but not in vertical width.

C. Mouth larger in vertical width but not in horizontal width.

A.   A mouth larger both in horizontal width and vertical height is the result of great overconsumption of carbohydrates and fats, including refined grains and flours, potatoes and fruits, sugar and vegetable-quality fats, during the embryonic and growing periods. This kind of mouth is often seen among people who have originated in a tropical climate, where these kinds of food are more likely to be eaten. In such cases, the peripheral parts of the body, such as the skin and muscles, appear stronger than average, while the internal organs such as the heart, liver, spleen and small intestine tend to be weaker, tending toward looseness. This is a generally yin type of constitution and condition.

B.   A mouth that is horizontally wider but normal in vertical height shows that the person has consumed, during the embryonic and growing periods, both animal-quality foods—such as meat, poultry, eggs and dairy products—and refined vegetable foods such as refined grains, flour products, sugar and fruits, and various soft drinks and beverages. Modern people have rapidly developed this type of mouth, which shows an unbalanced physical and mental constitution: physically, losing the ability of endurance and resistance, and mentally, losing the qualities of self-discipline and perseverance.

C.   A mouth larger in vertical height but not in horizontal width shows that the person has consumed excessive amounts of salts and other minerals (yang) together with dairy products, refined grains and flours, fruits and sugar, fat and oil, soft drinks and other beverages (yin). This type of mouth shows a general tendency toward chronic weakness of the digestive organs and functions. This condition also occurs in people who have received proper food during the embryonic period, but who consumed foods of more yin quality during the childhood growing period. We can say that this type of person is constitutionally yang but conditionally yin.

2.   *Special Characteristics*

Besides the general tendencies outlined above, there are a number of other conditions that show different characteristics, and these may change slowly or quickly according to changes in the environment and the kinds of foods and drinks consumed. The symptoms outlined below reflect these changing physical and mental conditions.

A.   The color of the lips changes according to fluctuations in blood quality and circulation. Various colors reflect different conditions:

Color	Condition
Pinkish red	Good blood quality and circulation. Respiratory, circulatory and digestive functions are normal and sound.
Vivid red	Blood capillaries are abnormally expanded, showing that the respiratory function is abnormal. Blood pressure tends to be higher and the speed of circulation tends to be faster. This color often appears in the lips when infections or inflammations are present.
White	Blood capillaries may be abnormally con-

Color	Condition
	stricted; or, there is a deficiency of hemoglobin; or, stagnation and slowness of blood circulation is taking place. Anemia, leukemia and other similar blood conditions often produce this lip color.
Dark	The blood plasma contains excessive salts and fatty acids, resulting in slowness and stagnation of blood circulation, as well as abnormal constriction of the blood capillaries. Disorders in kidney and urinary functions, and in liver and gallbladder functions are indicated.
Reddish dark	Excessive consumption of protein and saturated fats, together with excessive salts, often creates this color. It shows disorders in heart and circulatory functions, lung and respiratory functions, kidney and urinary functions, as well as disorders in the functions of the liver, gallbladder, spleen and pancreas.
Pinkish white	Excessive consumption of dairy products, fats, sugar and fruits often produces this color, indicating weakening lymphatic functions and hormonal disorders. Allergies, skin troubles, Hodgkin's disease, asthma and other similar circulatory, respiratory and hormonal disorders often show this color.
Purplish dark	Stagnation of blood circulation and serious malfunction of the blood cells, due to improper dietary practices and degeneration of the functions of such major organs as the intestines, liver, spleen, kidneys and lungs. This color is known as a sign that physical death is approaching.

B. *Abnormal colors* may also appear on certain areas of the lips for a relatively short time, indicating that abnormal conditions are present in certain parts of the body. For example:

Color	Condition
Yellowish shade	Due to the excessive consumption of poultry and eggs, dairy products—especially cheese—as well as other foods containing a large amount of saturated fats, the functions of the liver and gallbladder are in disorder.
Whitish patches	Excessive amounts of dairy foods and fats are being discharged. Temporary disorders in the digestive, respiratory, and lymphatic functions are indicated.
Black spots	Discharge of excessive carbohydrates, including refined sugar, honey, and fruit sugars. Disorders in the kidney and urinary functions are indicated. These spots also appear when hardened fats are accumulating in the digestive tract.
Dark reddish spots	Stagnation of blood circulation in the portion of the digestive vessel that corresponds to the area of the mouth where the spots appear.

C. Closed mouth and loose mouth. A mouth that is naturally closed (A), except when speaking or laughing, shows a generally sound nervous system and normal digestive and respiratory conditions (Fig. 25). However, a mouth that is tightly closed to an abnormal extent (B) indicates disorders in the liver, gallbladder, or kidneys due to the excessive intake of salts, meat,

Fig. 25   Forms of the Mouth: Looseness

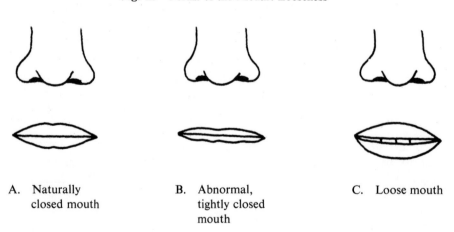

| A. Naturally closed mouth | B. Abnormal, tightly closed mouth | C. Loose mouth |

poultry, eggs and other animal foods. On the other hand, a loose mouth (C) shows disorders in the digestive, respiratory, and excretory functions, and also in the nervous functions, due to excessive consumption of raw vegetables, fruits, fruit juices, sugar and other sweetners, drugs and medications, as well as an overconsumption of food and drink in general.

D.   *Swollen lips* indicate digestive disorders (Fig. 26). A swollen and expanded upper lip indicates stomach trouble, including indigestion, due to the excessive intake of poor-quality foods. A swollen and expanded lower lip indicates intestinal troubles, including indigestion, gas production, constipation, and diarrhea. More than seven out of ten modern people suffer from at least one of these disorders, and their lower lips are far more expanded than their upper lips. If the swollen and expanded lower lip is also wet, the intestinal disorder is accompanied with diarrhea.

Fig. 26   Forms of the Mouth: Swollen Lips

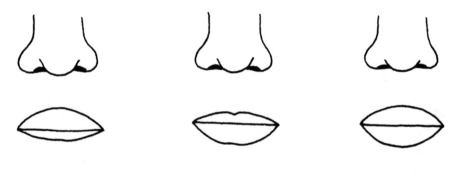

Upper lip swollen:
Stomach disorders

Lower lip swollen:
Intestinal disorders

Both lips swollen:
Both stomach and
intestinal disorders

Fig. 27   Mouth with Crust

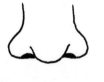

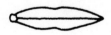

Crust formation at the corner
of the mouth.

E.   *Crust produced at the corners of the mouth* shows digestive trouble due to the excessive consumption of animal protein with oily and greasy foods (Fig. 27). This disorder occurs especially in the area of the duodenum. If the crust has a yellowish color, the excretion of bile from the liver and gallbladder is abnormal, due to the consumption of a large amount of saturated fats from foods such as meat, poultry, eggs, cheese, and fatty types of fish and seafood.

Fig. 28   Mouth with Vertical Wrinkles   Fig. 29   Edges of the Mouth

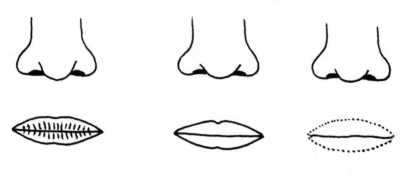

Vertical wrinkles on the lips   Clearly defined edges   Unclear edges

F.   Vertical wrinkles appearing on the lips show a recession of hormonal functions, especially of the gonad hormones, indicating that sexual functions are declining (Fig. 28). However, these wrinkles also appear in case of dehydration, caused by a lack of liquid or by the overconsumption of dry foods and salts.

G.   A mouth with a clearly-defined edge is the result of a proper volume of food and drink, and shows that the digestive system has a generally sound condition; while a mouth with an unclear edge is caused by the intake of an excessive amount of food and drink, showing weakness in the digestive and excretory functions (Fig. 29).

H.   The central part of the lips is clearly shaped if balanced foods, especially rich in minerals, were taken during the embryonic period (Fig. 30). Physically, this shows that the heart, small intestine and sexual ability are gen-

Fig. 30   Central Part of Lips

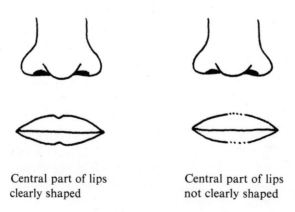

Central part of lips   Central part of lips
clearly shaped   not clearly shaped

erally sound; and mentally, it shows perseverance and a strong self-orienta-
tion. On the other hand, if the central part of the lips is not clearly formed,
it shows a native weakness in the heart, small intestine and sexual ability,
as well as in the stomach and pancreatic functions, including a tendency for
developing indigestion. In this case, a diabetic condition may also develop if
an excessive amount of sweetners, fruits and fatty foods are consumed over a
long time.

I. If the corners of the mouth appear like the angles of a square when the
mouth is wide open or laughing, it is traditionally called the "Devil's Mouth
(Fig. 31)." This type of mouth results from the overconsumption of animal
foods—especially less-cooked meat—and raw fruits during the embryonic and
early growing periods. It shows a mental tendency toward egocentric behavior.

Fig. 31 "Devil's Mouth"

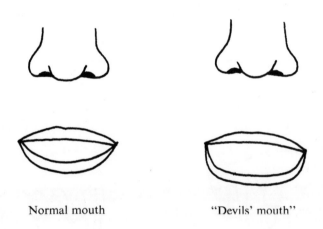

Normal mouth   "Devils' mouth"

The Teeth

During childhood we have 20 teeth, and as adults we have 32. The shape and
condition of our teeth shows the quality of the food consumed during their
growing period. Depending upon the volume and quality of food, the shape,
pattern, and even the number of teeth may vary. Following are guidelines for
diagnosis (see Fig. 32).

A. The number of teeth. Adults usually have 32 teeth: eight incisors, four
canines, eight premolars, and twelve molars. However, a full set of molars
does not grow normally unless a balanced diet has been eaten. Especially a
diet lacking in cereal grains can often result in the lack of the third molars
—the "wisdom teeth"—or, they may grow abnormally, producing pain or
deformation.

B.   Direction of growth.   Front teeth growing outward (a) show that excessive yin foods such as raw vegetables, fruits, and juices were eaten during a period of several years while the teeth were growing. On the other hand, teeth growing inward (b) show that more yang foods were eaten, including animal food, dry flour products, and more salty, over-cooked food. Teeth that are generally straight (c) and that bite together well show that the diet was well-balanced.

C.   Irregular growth.   Teeth growing in different directions—some pointing

Fig. 32   Forms of the Teeth

a.   Front teeth growing outward   b.   Teeth growing inward

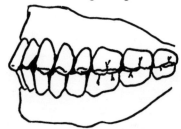 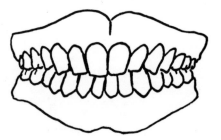

c.   Teeth growing generally straight

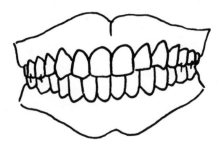 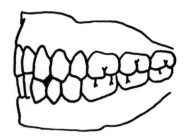

d.   Space between the teeth

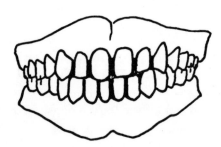 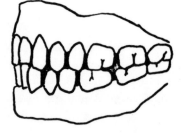

out, and some in—show that the diet during their growth was chaotic, with no regular pattern, resulting in a disharmonious physical and mental constitution. Those who have such irregular teeth are prone to frequent changes of mind and attitude.

D.   Spaces between the teeth (d. in Fig. 32) are caused by expansion of the jaws and gums, due to the overconsumption of yin foods. People with this condition often show a tendency to be scattered in their thinking and attitude. A space between the two major frontal incisors has been called traditionally "the sign of separation," or the sign of leaving the parents' home at an early age. Similarly, it has been said that such a person is unable to see his parents at the time of their death.

E.   Size of the teeth.   Larger teeth are the result of a comparatively yin diet, rich in protein and fat, while smaller teeth indicate that the diet was rich in carbohydrates and minerals.

F.   Abnormal tooth surface.   Vertical ridges on the tooth surface are due to the overconsumption of salts and carbohydrates, and a lack of protein and fat (Fig. 33). Teeth with small, pinhole-like dots also result from a lack of good-quality protein and fat and fresh vegetables, and an excess of salt and minerals. Serrated edges on the front teeth often result from the same cause.

Fig. 33   Abnormal Teeth

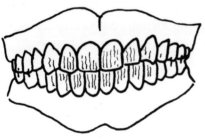

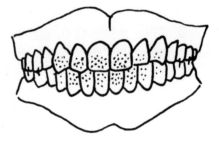

a.   Teeth with vertical ridges   b.   Teeth with small, pinhole-like dots

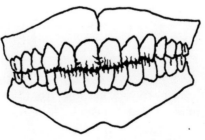

c.   Front teeth with serrated edges

G. *Tooth decay*, including cavities, root decay and loss of teeth, is caused by nutritional imbalance. Overconsumption of simple sugars and refined flour products is often the main cause, because these foods burn up minerals —including calcium—and some vitamins, when they enter the bloodstream.

Tooth decay arises symmetrically, generally affecting the teeth one-by-one in a distinct pattern. For example, if a tooth in the upper right jaw is decaying, the corresponding tooth in the upper left jaw is probably also decaying; or, the tooth immediately below on the lower right jaw is decaying. The 32 teeth correspond to the 32 vertebrae of the spine, and therefore to all major organs and glands. When teeth decay, therefore, it indicates that the corresponding major organs and glands are weakening. For example, some of the major tooth-organ correspondences are as follows:

Teeth	Organs and Functions
Incisors	Respiratory and circulatory organs and glands.
Canines	Liver, gallbladder, spleen, pancreas and stomach.
Premolars	Upper intestinal region; excretory system.
Molars	Lower digestive vessel, especially the small and large intestines; reproductive organs and glands.

H. *Color of the teeth.* Healthy teeth normally have a light ivory color. However, other colors are sometimes seen that indicate abnormal conditions, caused by smoking, drinking, and certain foods that have been eaten over a long period:

—*A light yellow color* may be the result of forgetting to brush the teeth, but a *deep yellow or dark brown color* is due to smoking habits.

—*A grey color* arises from a lark of fresh leafy vegetables, and may indicate disorders in the liver, gallbladder, spleen and pancreas and their functions.

—*A purplish color* is caused by the consumption of extremely yin foods such as certain fruits or juices, and shows a possible weakening in the respiratory functions.

I. *Teeth that chip easily* indicate an overconsumption of dry flour products and salt, especially when eaten after many years of sugar and milk consumption.

J. *Lack of normal growth of the teeth*, especially during childhood, arises not only from unbalanced nutrition, but also from the overconsumption of milk—even mothers' milk—for an unusually long period. Cows' milk and goats' milk weaken human teeth, and even human milk weakens the growing teeth if it is given beyond a reasonable period. When an infant begins to grow teeth, it is time for a reduction in breast-feeding and a gradual increase in soft baby food.

K.   Crooked teeth, which often create pressure on other teeth, are due to an abnormal diet, including the intake of excessive meat, poultry, eggs, dairy food and sugar, fruits, and soft drinks, and a lack of grains, beans, and vegetables.

The Gums and Mouth Cavity

A.   Swollen gums, often accompanied by pain and inflammation, are caused by the overconsumption of liquid, oil, sugar, fruits and juices.

B.   Receding gums are caused by either the overconsumption of yang foods—including animal food, salts, and dried food—or the overconsumption of yin foods, including sugar, honey, chocolate, soft drinks, fruits and juices.

C.   Abnormally red or purple gums that are not swollen are caused by a combination of yang animal food or salts and yin sugar, fruits, juices, soft drinks and chemicals. Similar colors accompanied by swollenness are caused by the overconsumption of yin foods and drinks.

D.   Pale, whitish gums indicate poor circulation as well as a lack of hemoglobin in the bloodstream, due to anemia caused by nutritional imbalance.

E.   Pimples appearing on the inner wall of the mouth cavity are eliminations of one or all of the following: excessive protein, fat and oil from both animal and vegetable sources, sugar and sugar products.

F.   Bleeding gums, in most cases, are caused by broken blood capillaries which have been weakened by a lack of salt and other minerals in the bloodstream. In rare cases, they can also be caused by overconsumption of animal food, dry flour products, salts and minerals, and a lack of fresh vegetables and fruits, as in the case of scurvy.

G.   Inflammation deep in the throat, with or without swolleness of the tonsils, is caused by the overconsumption of yin foods, including fruits, juices, sugar, soda, icy cold drinks, as well as milk, as in the case of tonsilitis. If the condition is accompanied by white patches deep in the throat, the same cause is indicated, together with the overconsumption of animal fat, including the fats in meat, poultry and eggs, and all dairy food, as in the case of diphtheria.

The Tongue and Uvula

The tongue and uvula also show the physical and mental constitution and the current condition (Fig. 34).

Fig. 34   Forms of the Tongue

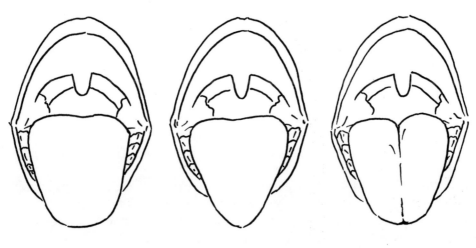

a.   Wide tongue with   b.   Narrow tongue with   c.   Tongue with a divided
     a round tip   a sharp, pointed tip   tip

A.   *The shape of the tongue* varies from person to person:

—*A wide tongue with a round tip* results when the mother eats food of vegetable quality during pregnancy. The physiological and psychological conditions of such a person are generally harmonious, gentle and understanding.

—*A narrow tongue with a sharp, pointed tip* is caused by heavy consumption of animal quality food during the time of pregnancy. A person with this kind of tongue tends to be physically rigid and tight, and mentally aggressive and offensive, with a narrow mind.

—*A tongue with a divided tip* is caused by the frequent consumption of raw animal and vegetable foods during the embryonic period, and shows a tendency to be indecisive and changeable.

—*A flat tongue* comes from grain and vegetable consumption during embryonic and early childhood growth, and shows a tendency to be harmonious with the environment.

—*A thick tongue* is caused by overconsumption of animal food, protein and fat during the period of embryonic and childhood growth, and shows a more active, offensive and aggressive character.

Fig. 35 Areas on Tongue Corresponding to Internal Organs

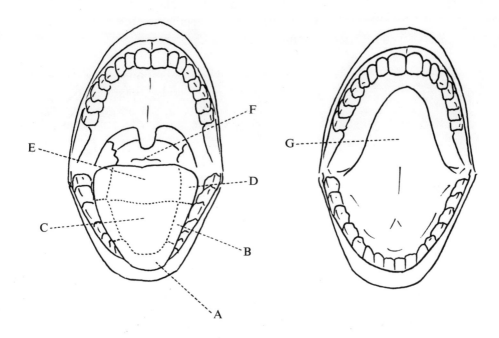

Top and underside of the tongue

B. The tongue represents the whole digestive vessel, and each area of the tongue corresponds to a certain region of the digestive vessel (see Fig. 35):

—*The tip area (A)* corresponds to the rectum and descending colon of the large intestine.

—*The peripheral area (B)* corresponds to the large intestine.

—*The middle region (C)* corresponds to the small intestine.

—*The back edge region (D)* corresponds to the duodenum, liver, gall-bladder, and pancreas.

—*The near back region (E)* corresponds to the stomach.

—*The back region (F, the "root of the tongue")* corresponds to the esophagus.

—*The underside (G)* reflects the condition of the blood and lymph circulation in each corresponding area.

C. The color of the upper side of the tongue. According to the corresponding areas outlined above, a change of color in any region shows an abnormal condition in the corresponding organ or region:

Color	Condition
Dark red	Inflammation, ulcer, or cancer.
White	Stagnation of blood circulation; accumulation of fat and mucus; anemia; or lack of hemoglobin.
Yellow color and coating	Inflammation and over-secretion due to excessive bile from the liver and gallbladder. Accumulation of fat, mainly from poultry, eggs and dairy food.
White patches	Elimination of dairy food or fat and oil from both animal and vegetable sources. General tiredness of the digestive functions.
Blue, purple:	Overconsumption of yin foods, including fruits, juices, soft drinks, chemicals, drugs and medications, as well as sugar.

D. *The color of the underside of the tongue*

Color	Condition
Excessive red color	Inflammation, excess liquid, or excess hemoglobin in the bloodsteam due to the overconsumption of liquid, fruits, juices and animal food.
Excessive blue and green	Disorders in the blood vessels due to the overconsumption of animal fat, dairy food, fruits, juices and sugar.
Excessive yellow	Inflammation or stagnation of fat and mucus due to excessive bile secretion or the consumption of dairy food, poultry and eggs.
Excessive purple	Disorders in the blood vessels and lymphatic stream due to the overconsumption of sugar, fruits, juices, chemicals, drugs and medications.

E. *Pimples on the tongue* are also caused by the elimination of excessive protein, fat, or sugar from both animal and vegetable sources. They often arise from a combination of fish and fruits, meat and vegetable oil, flour and dairy food, eggs and citrus juices.

2. The Eyes and Eyebrows

The Eyebrows

The eyebrows reflect the nervous, digestive, respiratory, circulatory and excretory systems, and therefore they reveal the constitution developed during the period of pregnancy, as well as the current condition.

The eyebrows as a whole show the history of a person's development during pregnancy. The inner portion of the brows reflects the early embryonic stage; the middle portion shows the middle stage; and the ends of the brows reflect the last stage of pregnancy (Fig. 36). Since the course of life after birth generally repeats the growing process that took place during pregnancy, these sections of the eyebrows also show respectively the youth, middle age and old of a person's entire lifetime.

Fig. 36   Areas of the Eyebrows

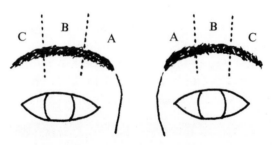

Left eyebrow—More paternal influence
Right eyebrow—More maternal influence

A—Early part of pregnancy; youth
B—Middle part of pregnancy; middle age
C—Late part of pregnancy; old age

By examining the eyebrows, we can diagnose general constitutional and conditional characteristics as follows.

1.   The space between the eyebrows

The space between the eyebrows is a result of the eating habits of the mother during pregnancy, especially during the third and fourth months. A smaller space is caused by the consumption of excessive animal food, especially meat, poultry, eggs, fish and caviar, as well as over-cooked vegetables flavored with large amounts of salt (Fig. 37). On the other hand, a wider space between the eyebrows is caused by the mother's consumption of milk, sugar, fruits, soft drinks, and raw leafy vegetables, as well as vegetables of tropical origin.

Fig. 37   Space between the Eyebrows

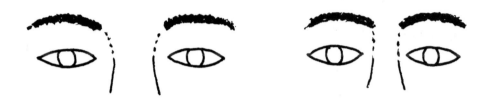

Wider space between the eyebrows   Narrower space between the eyebrows

A shorter distance between the eyebrows shows a general tendency for such organs as the liver, pancreas, kidneys, heart, and other yang, compacted organs and glands to be easily affected with disorders, as a result of the excessive intake of yang food during the growing period. A wider distance between the brows, on the other hand, indicates that disorders may arise in such organs as the lungs, intestines, bladder and gallbladder, because of an excessive consumption of yin food during the growing period. Mentally, the shorter distance shows a more narrow mind, stubborn determination, and emotional sharpness, while the wider distance shows uncertainty, insecurity, indecisiveness, and lack of determination. A distinctly wide space between the brows has been traditionally called "the sign of a widow," or a sign of separation.

2.   The angle of the eyebrows

The angle of the brows also shows the physical and mental constitution, and is also caused by the food the mother ate during pregnancy (Fig. 38):

A.   Upward-slanting eyebrows are formed by the consumption of excessive animal food, and represent a more aggressive and offensive character. Susceptibility to liver and heart trouble is indicated.

B.   Downward-slanting eyebrows are caused by low animal food consumption and more food of vegetable quality, showing a gentle and understanding character, with a potential for kidney and intestinal troubles.

Fig. 38 Angle of the Eyebrows

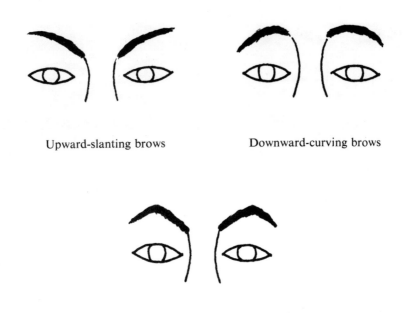

Upward-slanting brows   Downward-curving brows

Peaked brows

As a general tendency, animal-caused eyebrows indicate a shorter life expectancy, while vegetable-caused brows show the potential for a longer life.

C. An orderly, balanced angle—smooth, curving eyebrows—is created by well-balanced food consumed by the mother during pregnancy, and shows physical and mental balance.

D. Peaked eyebrows whose inner portion slants upward while the outer portion curves downward show that animal food was heavily consumed during the first part of pregnancy, and more vegetable food was consumed in the latter part of pregnancy. A person with this type of eyebrows has a general tendency to be active physically and socially but gentle and sometimes timid in mentality. During youth, he is more physically and socially active, but in the latter part of his life he is occupied with more mental and spiritual matters. In this case, the kidneys, liver, and spleen are easily affected by both excessively yin and yang foods.

3. The condition of the hair in the eyebrows

A. The thickness of the hairs shows the degree of vitality. The denser the eyebrows, the more energetic a person is; the thinner, the less energetic (Fig. 39).

Fig. 39   Various Kinds of Eyebrows

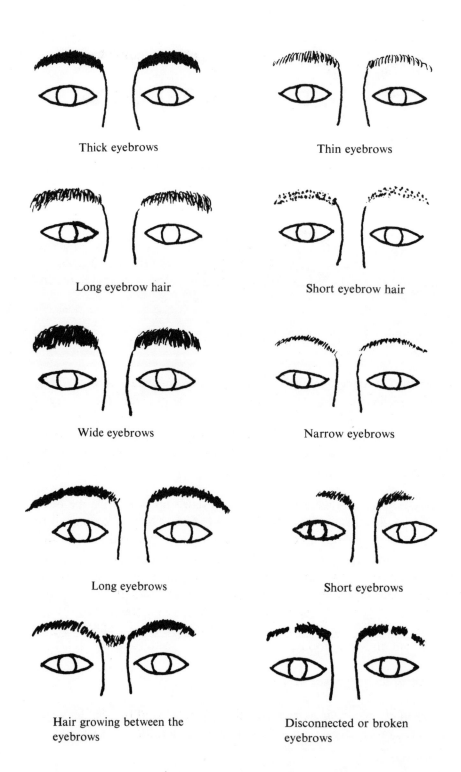

Thick eyebrows

Thin eyebrows

Long eyebrow hair

Short eyebrow hair

Wide eyebrows

Narrow eyebrows

Long eyebrows

Short eyebrows

Hair growing between the
eyebrows

Disconnected or broken
eyebrows

B. Longer hairs in the brows show a more mentally and spiritually active character, while *shorter hairs* show a more physically active character.

C. Broad, full eyebrows show active vitality, and narrow eyebrows show less vitality. If the eyebrows are becoming narrower, it indicates physical and mental degeneration.

D. Long eyebrows indicate a long life; *short eyebrows*, a shorter life. (Compare with the life lines on the palm.) If the eyebrows are becoming shorter, physical degeneration is taking place and serious malfunctions in the major organs are progressing.

E. When the eyebrow hair changes color, it indicates a substantial change in physical and mental condition. When the eyebrows change from a normal dark color to grey or white, it is due either to advancing age or to the eating of excessive salt and minerals. If the eyebrow hair changes to a lighter color, it is caused by the excessive intake of more minerals and animal food, while a change toward a darker color is caused by eating more vegetable-quality food.

F. Hair growing between the brows is caused by the intake of dairy food and fatty animal food during the third and fourth months of pregnancy. If a person has this type of eyebrows, his liver, pancreas, and spleen tend to be easily affected by the consumption of excessive amounts of animal food and oily or fatty foods, including dairy products.

G. Broken or disconnected brows indicate the possibility of developing a a serious sickness at some time in life. (Compare with a broken life line on the palm.)

The Eyes

The eyes represent the entire physical, mental and spiritual condition. The eyes are one of our most expressive instruments, showing physical, mental and spiritual change. The eyes tell everything!

1. The distance between the eyes.

A. A shorter distance, as in the case of the eyebrows, results from a strongly yang quality of food eaten during the early part of pregnancy, and indicates a more aggressive, narrow-minded and stubborn but emotionally and intellectually sharp character (Fig. 40). There is a potential for the organs in the middle region of the body, such as the liver, pancreas, spleen and kidneys, to easily become out of order through the intake of excessive animal-

Fig. 40   Distance between the Eyes

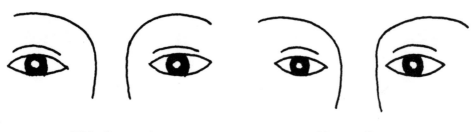

Wide distance   Narrow distance

quality food.

B.   A wider distance between the eyes, on the other hand, results from a more yin quality of food, including salad, sugars, soft drinks, and fruits, and indicates a more loose, indecisive, slow, but gentle character. The organs in the middle region of the body named above have a tendency to be easily affected by an excess of yin foods, including sugars, soft drinks, tropical fruits, and aromatic, stimulant foods and beverages.

2.   The angle of the eyes

A.   Eyes that slant upward at the outer edge result from the mother's intake of well-cooked and well-salted grains and vegetables during the time of pregnancy, and indicate a tendency toward clear emotional and intellectual character (Fig. 41).

B.   Eyes that slant downward at the ends, on the other hand, are caused by the mother's intake of less-cooked, less-salted vegetable-quality foods, including fruits and fruit juice, during pregnancy, and indicate a more gentle and accepting character.

Fig. 41   Angle of the Eyes

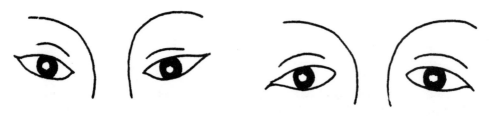

Eyes slanting up   Eyes slanting down

Fig. 42   Size of the Eyes

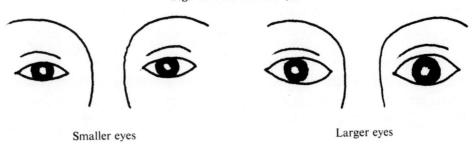

Smaller eyes   Larger eyes

3.   Size of the eyes

A.   Small eyes are caused by yang foods, including well-cooked vegetable and animal quality foods, consumed not only during the time of pregnancy, but also during the childhood growing period (Fig. 42). They show a more determined, active and self confident character, together with physical strength, vitality and endurance. If the eyes are abnormally small, they show a tendency toward a sharp, aggressive character.

B.   Large eyes, on the other hand, are caused by the intake of yin foods such as less-cooked and raw vegetables, fruits and fruit juice, and indicate a more mentally sensitive, delicate and gentle character. Abnormally large eyes indicate nervous disorders, including extra sensitivity, irritability, nervousness, timidity and lack of confidence.

Generally speaking, it is desirable for men to have eyes that are smaller and narrower, and for women to have more open and round eyes.

4.   The eyelids and eyelashes

A.   Single, tight eyelids result from the consumption of well-cooked grains and vegetables during the time of pregnancy, and show a general tendency toward mental clarity (Fig. 43).

Fig. 43   The Eyelids

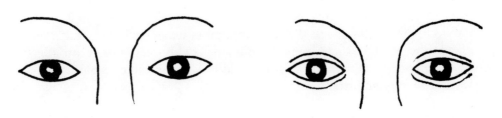

Single and tight eyelids   Double and loose eyelids

B. *Double, loose eyelids* result from the mother's intake of a large volume of fats and fluids during pregnancy, and often represent physical strength. However, eyelids that are swollen and red or purple indicate a current excessive intake of fruits, sugar and other sweets, soda, soft drinks, vegetables of tropical origin, and various alcoholic beverages and stimulants. This condition can also show an intake of drugs and medications. General weakness in the digestive functions, and abnormal sensitivity of the nervous functions are indicated. The organs mainly affected are the kidneys, intestines, spleen, liver, and reproductive organs, as well as the hormonal functions.

C. *"The Eyes of the Phoenix."* The area of the lower eyelid indicated in Fig. 44 as area "x" varies according to the constitution developed in the mother's womb. If area "x" is flat and clear, it is traditionally known as "The Eyes of the Phoenix," and is considered a sign of leadership. However, if there is no area "x" or if that area is swollen, it indicates a lack of clear judgement.

Fig. 44   The Eyelids

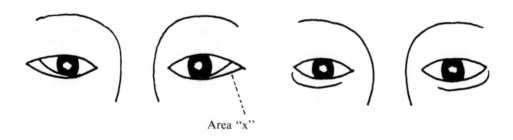

Area "x"

"The Eyes of the Phoenix"   Swollen eyelids

D. *Blinking.* The frequency of blinking is lower in children, whose constitutions are more yang, strong and active, and it increases as we approach adulthood. On the average, a healthy adult blinks about once every 20 seconds, or three times per minute. A person who blinks much less is currently in a more active, sharp condition, in both physical and mental character. A person who blinks more than three times per minute is in a state of declining health, due to the consumption of excessive liquid, fruit, sugar and other yin foods and drinks. If blinking is abnormally frequent, a person is suffering from nervous disorders and is experiencing extreme sensitivity, fear, timidity and irritability.

E. *Long eyelashes* indicate the intake of excessive liquid, raw vegetables and fruits, and other yin foods (Fig. 45).

Fig. 45   Various Kinds of Eyelashes

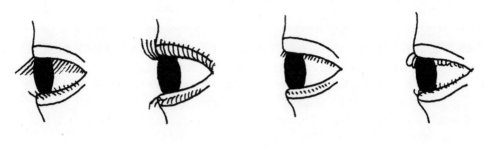

Long eyelashes   Curving outward   Shorter eyelashes   Curving inward

F.   If the eyelashes curve outward, it shows abnormal nervous sensitivity, and indicates that the reproductive functions are in a state of degeneration due to the consumption of excessive yin foods such as fruits, fruit juice, wine, sugar, sweets, soft drinks, aromatic stimulant foods and beverages as well as drugs and medications, during early childhood.

G.   Shorter eyelashes result from the intake of a more yang quality of food, including well-cooked salty food, roasted and baked food, and cooked animal food, and less intake of grain and vegetables.

H.   Eyelashes that curve inward indicate the excessive intake of strongly yang foods such as a large amount of salt, meat, eggs, fish, caviar, and poultry, without enough grains and vegetables to balance them. In this case, the reproductive functions are often abnormal, especially in women, who may experience menstrual cramps or lack of menstruation due to contraction of the ovaries.

5.   Change of color around the eyes

The colors around the eyes vary according to different physical and mental conditions, and change daily according to our daily health:

A.   Clear, clean, natural skin color.   This color shows sound physical and mental health, the result of proper diet and way of life. The physical and mental functions are operating harmoniously.

B.   Dark color.   This color arises when there is an excessively yang condition, including contraction of the kidneys and exhaustion of the adrenal and gonad hormones. Therefore, this color can appear due to the intake of excessive salt and roasted, baked, or dried foods. It often arises after excessive sexual intercourse, especially in people whose kidneys and excretory functions are weak. It also indicates stagnated metabolism in the kidneys and excretory system, and in the ovaries, testicles and reproductive functions.

C. *Reddish color.* This color appears when the blood capillaries are expanded from the intake of excessive yin foods and drinks, including liquids, fruits, juice, sugars, and many others, showing that the heart and circulatory system are now overworking. Redness on the eyelids may appear from time to time and shows an extreme state of the above condition, together with nervousness. This may arise among some women whose menstrual periods are irregular, when the period is due. However, if this condition continues chronically, the mental condition will become extremely nervous.

D. *Purplish color.* This color shows a more advanced stage of the condition described above under "reddish color," and is caused mainly by the consumption of drugs, chemicals, medications, refined simple sugars and other extremely yin foods and drinks. The nervous system, circulatory system and excretory system are all in disorder. People who have this color around the eyes usually experience hallucinations, and feel cold at the peripheral parts of the body such as the hands and feet.

E. *Yelllowish color.* This color appears when the liver and gallbladder are over-functioning. It can be caused by eating too much cheese and other dairy products, and also by an excessive intake of certain root vegetables such as carrots, and some round vegetables such as pumpkin and squash. It can also show a temporary disorder of the kidneys and excretory functions.

F. *Greyish color.* A greyish, pale color appears in cases of malfunction of the kidneys and sometimes the lungs, mainly because of metabolic stagnation due to the excessive intake of heavy, fatty, animal food, and the over-consumption of salt and other yang foods. This color also indicates that the endocrine and lymph systems are not functioning properly, especially in the regions of the respiratory and reproductive organs. An imbalance of minerals in the bloodstream, which arises not only from improper food and drink, but also from improper environmental air conditions, can produce this color.

6. *Pimples appearing around the eyes*

Pimples are the body's attempt to eliminate certain food substances that have been consumed in excess. They can appear in various areas around the eyes:

A. *Pimples above the eyelid and below the eyebrows* are eliminations of mucus, fat and oil, caused by the excessive intake of oil, sugar, and dairy products. If the pimples are also yellow in color, the diet has included poultry, eggs, and/or cheese, as well.

B. *Pimples on the eyelid* are eliminations of protein, fat, and sugar, caused by the overconsumption of animal food and fruits. The consumption of oily fish, oranges or other fruits and juices can often produce reddish pimples near the corner of the eyelid.

C. *Pimples below the lower eyelid* are eliminations of both protein and sugar, caused by the consumption of excessive fatty meat and sugar, or fruit juice. Whitish-yellow pimples in this area show the consumption of eggs, dairy products and other animal fats.

While these eliminations are proceeding in the form of pimples in the different areas near the eyes, the kidneys and excretory system, and the spleen and lymphatic system are temporarily affected by this excessive intake of unnecessary foods and drinks. If the pimples itch and are inflamed, the process of elimination is going on very actively, but if they have no itching and inflammation, the elimination is proceeding gradually.

7. *Eyebags*

During adulthood, but increasingly even during youth in the modern age, many people develop eyebags under the lower eyelid (Fig. 46). Eyebags may have one of two causes, although the appearance may be similar:
(1) eyebags due to a pool of liquid, and (2) eyebags due to pooled mucus. The first type of eyebag appears watery and swollen, and the second type appears more fatty and swollen.

Fig. 46   Eyebags

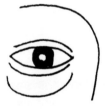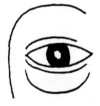

Very swollen eyebags

Both types of eyebags show disorders of the kidney, bladder, and excretory functions. Especially the first type of eyebag indicates swollenness of the kidney tissues and frequent urination due to the excessive intake of liquid of any kind, including all sorts of beverages, fruits and juices.

The second type of eyebag does not necessarily demonstrate frequent urination, but shows mucus and fat accumulation in the kidney tissues. If small pimples or small dark spots appear on these mucus-caused eyebags, it shows that the accumulated mucus and fat in the kidney tissues is forming kidney stones. If these eyebags are chronic, mucus accumulation is developing in the ureter, the wall of the bladder, the ovaries, Fallopian tubes and uterus, and in and around the prostate glands, creating bacterial activity, inflammation, itching, vaginal discharge, ovarian cysts, and eventually the growth of tumors and cancer in these areas.

Both types of eyebags also indicate the decline of physical and mental vitality as a natural result of the above conditions. Tiredness, overloaded body systems, fatigue, laziness, forgetfulness, indecisiveness and loss of clear judgement are developing.

The water-caused eyebag is easily corrected by the restriction of liquid intake, while the mucus-caused eyebag can be corrected by the restriction of all mucus- and fat-forming food, including especially dairy products, meat fat, poultry, sugars, refined flour, and all sorts of oil, although it takes much longer than in the case of the first type of eyebag.

8. The pink area inside the lower eyelids

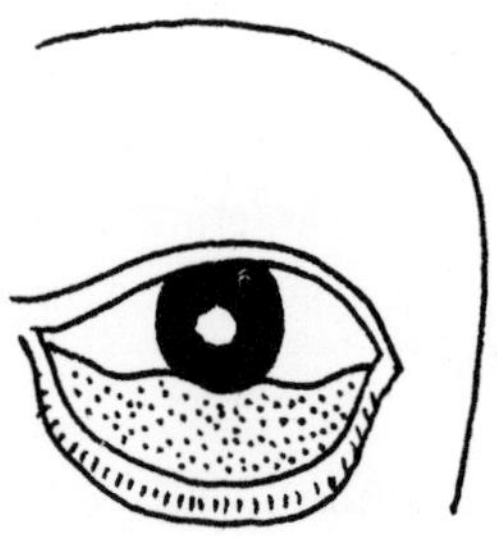

This area shows mainly the circulatory condition (Fig. 47). Variations in color indicate different conditions, as follows:

Fig. 47   Inside of Lower Eyelid

A. Light pink color with a smooth surface indicates a healthy, normal circulatory condition.

B. Red color with expanded capillaries indicates high blood pressure or excretory disorders, due to the excessive intake of yin foods, especially liquids, alcohol, fruits, juices and sugars. It also shows inflammation of the circulatory system, and nervousness.

C. A whitish color shows an anemic condition, caused by the excessive intake of yin foods. It can sometimes be caused by yang food including salt and roasted or baked flour products. Often a condition of leukemia shows this color.

D. A reddish-yellow color is caused by the consumption of excess yang, animal food including poultry, eggs, and dairy products as well as excess yin foods including sugar, fruits, and others. This color shows disorders in the heart and circulatory system, together with disorders in the liver, spleen, and pancreas functions.

The Eyeball, Iris and White

The eyeballs are part of the nervous system, but they represent very well the whole physical and mental condition.

1. The size of the eyeballs

The eyeballs change in size due to the kinds of foods and drinks consumed, as well as according to age. During infancy and early childhood, the eyeballs are comparatively small, and they expand rapidly as growth progresses (Fig. 48). In general, between puberty and menopause, the size of the eyeballs stays fairly constant, with slight fluctuations due to changes in food and drink. Toward the end of life, after menopause, the eyeballs tend to contract, usually resulting in changes in sight.

Fig. 48   Size of the Eyeball

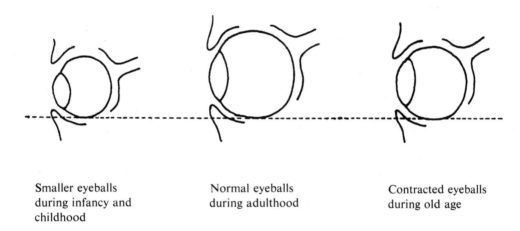

Smaller eyeballs
during infancy and
childhood

Normal eyeballs
during adulthood

Contracted eyeballs
during old age

A. Abnormal eyeball expansion caused by excess yin foods and drinks produces myopia, or nearsightedness (Fig. 49).

Fig. 49   Expansion and Contraction of the Eyeball and Lens

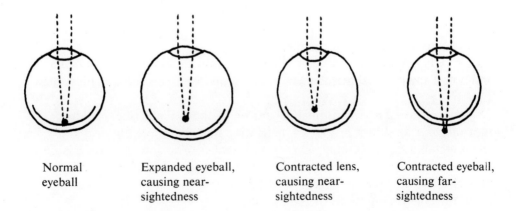

Normal
eyeball

Expanded eyeball,
causing near-
sightedness

Contracted lens,
causing near-
sightedness

Contracted eyeball,
causing far-
sightedness

B. Abnormal contraction of the lens of the eye caused by dehydration, excessive intake of salt, meat, and other animal food, also produces nearsightedness.

C. Abnormal contraction of the eyeball caused by dehydration, aging, excessive intake of yang foods including salt, dried foods, and animal food, produces farsightedness.

2. *Sanpaku*

Furthermore, abnormal expansion and contraction of the eyeballs produces a condition known as *sanpaku,* a Japanese word meaning "three whites," indicating that the eyeball has taken an abnormally high or low position (Fig. 50).

Fig. 50 Sanpaku Conditions

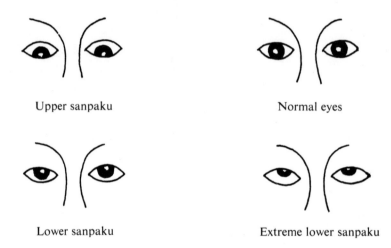

Upper sanpaku   Normal eyes

Lower sanpaku   Extreme lower sanpaku

A. Upper sanpaku. Contracted eyeballs, which are normal in infants and young children, produce upper *sanpaku* as illustrated in Fig. 50. However, if this condition continues beyond early childhood, or if it begins at a later age, it is a sign of abnormal mentality and behavior, including aggressiveness, violence, and uncontrollable passions.

After early childhood, through old age, a person should have no *sanpaku* condition if the physical metabolism is sound and well-balanced, as illustrated.

B. Lower sanpaku. Abnormal expansion of the eyeballs often produces lower *sanpaku,* as shown in Fig. 50, indicating that the whole physical and mental metabolism is becoming slower and weaker. This lower *sanpaku* is on the increase among modern people due to overconsumption of yin foods, although there are some instances of lower *sanpaku* caused by overconsumption of extremely yang foods including salt.

This condition also shows that the nerve cells of the brain are expanded, often resulting in abnormal thinking and behavior, which may lead to a fatal destiny. Those who commit crimes and treachery, those who are suspicious, and those who are the object of misunderstanding, attacks, or assassinations usually have this lower *sanpaku* condition. Extreme lower *sanpaku* indicates that death is drawing near. This condition appears universally in people who are going to meet death unexpectedly in the near future.

It is interesting to note that most criminals posted publicly as "Wanted" have either upper or lower *sanpaku*, and nearly all people who have been assassinated have had lower *sanpaku*, including Julius Caesar, Abraham Lincoln, Adolf Hitler, Mahatma Gandhi, John F. Kennedy, Robert F. Kennedy, and Martin Luther King.

In order to diagnose an lower *sanpaku* condition, ask the person to look up at a 45-degree angle. If white is showing beneath the iris, he or she already has lower *sanpaku*.

3. Wet eyeballs

Constant tear production, which is usually accompanied by many red, expanded capillaries on the white of the eye, often indicates glaucoma, and in some cases, detachment of the retina. This condition is caused by an excessive intake of liquids, juices, fruits and other watery foods.

4. The iris

The color of the iris differs according to the biological constitution which was developed from the time of conception by dietary practices and environmental conditions. Usually, people think that differences in the color of the iris occur because of racial differences, but actually they are the result of traditional ways of living.

A. *A light iris*, for example blue, shows that the person has originated in a more northern region where he has received less sunlight.

B. *A brown iris* is produced by a four-season climate.

C. *A dark iris* such as dark brown or black generally develops in a sunny, tropical environment.

The color of the iris has a tendency to change slightly throughout life— during infancy and childhood, darker; toward adulthood, lighter.

D. *Iridology*, or diagnosis according to observation of the iris, can reveal various physical and mental conditions. According to a study introduced by Dr. Bernard Jensen, Fig. 51 shows the general areas corresponding to various parts of the body.

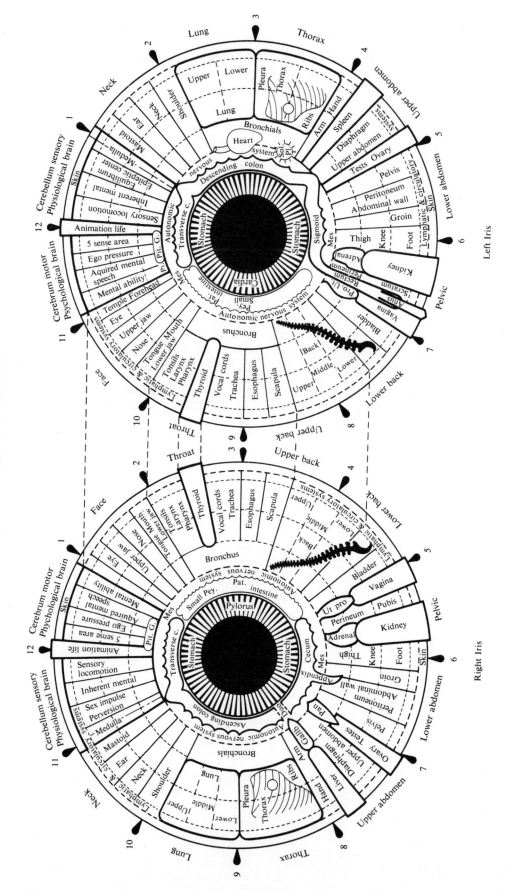

Fig. 51 Iridology by Bernard Jensen

5. The pupil

The condition of the pupil reflects very clearly the functions of the autonomic nerves. The pupil opens and closes according to the degree of brightness in the environment. The brighter the environment, the smaller the pupil becomes; the darker the environment, the larger the pupil. The speed of the autonomic reflex action shows the alertness of the autonomic nerves.

   A.   A pupil larger than average shows degeneration of the autonomic nerves, especially the parasympathetic nervous functions, due to an excessive consumption of yin foods and drinks as well as drugs, some vitamins and medications. Extreme dilation of the pupil arises at death. A large pupil accordingly indicates general degeneration and weakening of the physical and mental functions. Fear, nervousness, anxiety, and other mental disorders also arise when the pupils are enlarged.

   B.   A pupil smaller than average indicates healthy, sound physical and mental functions, mainly developed by eating grains and vegetables. Vitality, endurance, patience, perseverance, and resistance, both physically and mentally, are indicated. This condition in a person over the age of 60 shows potential longevity and good coordination among the major organs and glands.

   C.   A white, mucous cloud covering the pupil is a sign that cataracts are developing, due to the overconsumption of dairy products and other fats, together with sugar and sweets.

6. The white of the eye

As in the case of the iris, the white of the eye represents various parts of the whole body, as follows (see Fig. 52):

Area of the White	*Part of the Body*
Upper area ($\triangledown$)	Upper part of the body, including the brain, face, neck, chest, lungs, heart, and the upper spine.
Middle area ($\bigcirc$)	Middle region of the body, including the stomach, duodenum, spleen, pancreas, liver, gallbladder, kidneys, and middle spine.
Lower area ($\triangle$)	Lower region of the body, including the small and large intestines, bladder, reproductive organs, buttocks and lower region of the spine.

Fig. 52   Major Areas of the White of the Eye

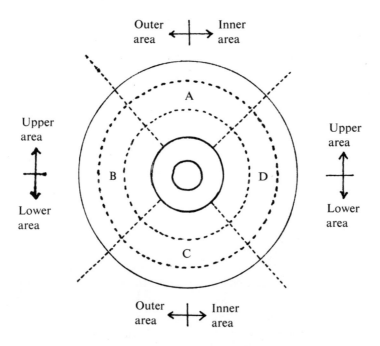

A—Upper regions of body
B—Middle front regions of body
C—Lower regions of body
D—Middle back regions of body

Outer dotted circle area—Digestive and
   respiratory functions
Inner dotted circle area—Circulatory and
   excretory functions
Iris and pupil—Nervous functions

Inner part of white—More compacted organs in each region
Outer part of white—More expanded organs in each region

Area of the White
Outside (▽)

Part of the Body
The front of the body, including the face,
forebrain, neck and chest, respiratory and
digestive systems and their connected organs
and glands.

Inside (△)

The back of the body, including the small
brain, neck, shoulders, spinal cord and connected tissues, waist, buttocks, and cervical
region.

Certain colors and marks appearing on the white of the eye indicate abnormal conditions in the corresponding areas of the body, as follows (see
Fig. 53):

Fig. 53   Marks on the White of the Eye

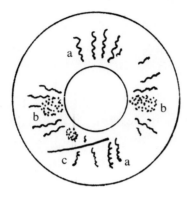 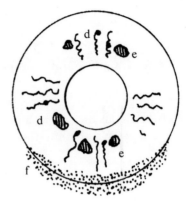

a—Expanded blood capillaries
b—White mucus patches
c—Straight long red line

d—Red spots—blood clots
e—Dark spots
f—Mucus under the eyeball

A.   A yellow color often seen in the peripheral part of the white shows an accumulation of fat and mucus caused by animal-quality food, indicating that the liver, gallbladder and digestive functions are in disorder.

B.   A grey or dark color sometimes seen in the middle and inner regions of the white indicates stagnation of the functions of the organs and glands, including disorders in the digestive, respiratory and lymphatic functions.

C.   A transparent or pale white color shows the presence of stagnated fat and mucus which may be progressing toward the growth of cysts, tumors and cancer. Disorders in the hormonal and lymphatic functions are indicated.

D.   A red color caused by many expanded blood capillaries indicates disorders in the circulatory and respiratory functions, caused by excessive consumption of yin foods and drinks. Menstrual irregularity and epileptic disorders are also reflected in various minute, expanded capillaries in the corresponding areas of the white.

E.   A straight, long red line in a certain part of the white often indicates abnormal deformation of blood vessels or tissues and muscles, which may be caused by a shock, accident or surgery in the corresponding area of the body.

F.   Red spots appearing here and there on the white show that blood clots or circulatory stagnation are arising in the organs, glands or muscles in the corresponding areas of the body.

G.   Dark spots appearing here and there on the white are an indication of the formation of fat deposits, cysts, tumors, and sometimes cancer, as well as stones and calcification in the corresponding areas of the body.

   H.   White mucous patches usually arising in the middle or lower part of the white indicate heavy fat accumulation, which is progressing toward the formation of cysts, tumors and cancer.

   I.   Mucus appearing at the lower part of the white, below the eyeball, is an indication of mucus and fat accumulation in the lower part of the body, including in and around the intestines, ovaries, uterus, Fallopian tubes, and prostate glands.

   J.   A cloudy white color with a grey tone covering most of the white signals a developing hardness of the eyeballs, caused by the excessive intake of fats with sugar, fruits and juices.

7.   The inside of the eyelids

Fig. 54   The area Inside the Upper and Lower Eyelids

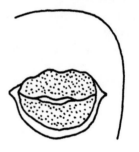

The areas inside the upper and lower eyelids are usually pink and have a smooth surface, under healthy conditions (Fig. 54). When the following changes develop in this area, certain disorders are shown:

   A.   Reddish color: This color shows expansion of the blood capillaries caused by excess yin foods, and indicates that reproductive, digestive and circulatory disorders may be developing.

   B.   A reddish-yellow color: Expansion of the blood capillaries is indicated, along with stagnation of fat and mucus, caused by the overconsumption of both yin foods and yang animal protein and fats, leading to disorders of the heart, liver, kidneys, and other major organs.

   C.   A white color: Lack of hemoglobin or blood circulation—overall anemia—caused mainly by the overconsumption of either extremely yang foods such as salt and dry flour products, or extremely yin foods including fruit juice, soft drinks, drugs, and chemicals.

   D.   Small dot-like pimples: These show the elimination of animal protein and saturated fat coming from meat, eggs, dairy products, fish and seafood which have been eaten to excess. If these pimples develop a red, inflamed condition, it is known as *trachoma.*

E. Large pimples: Usually one or two in number and with combined red, yellow and white colors, these show the elimination of animal protein and fats, vegetable oils, sugar, and excessive liquid.

3. The Nose, Cheeks and Ears

The Nose

The nose reflects the condition of the nervous system, the circulatory system, and certain functions of the digestive system. The type of nose, size, shape, color and other characteristics reveal specific conditions, as described below.

1. General characteristics

The shape of the nose corresponds to the size, quality and condition of the brain.

A. Type of nose. A well-formed nose with average length and roundness shows a balanced mentality, and a straight and longer nose shows a more sensitive nervous quality (Fig. 55). A short, flatter nose shows a tendency

Fig. 55 Forms of the Nose (1)

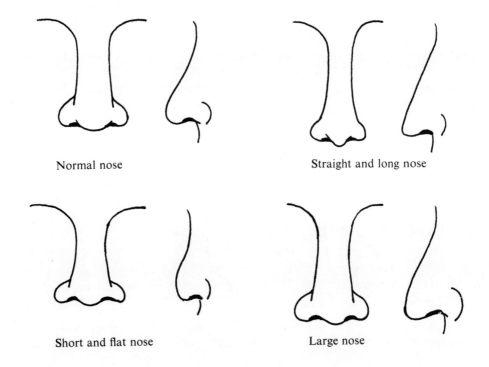

Normal nose

Straight and long nose

Short and flat nose

Large nose

toward determination and rigidity in thinking, while a larger nose, if not abnormally large, shows a larger thinking capacity.

B. *The sides of the nose.* The raised, bony areas on the sides of the nose indicate obscure thinking, while if these areas are less prominent, there is more of a tendency toward clear thinking (Fig. 56).

Fig. 56 Forms of the Nose (2)

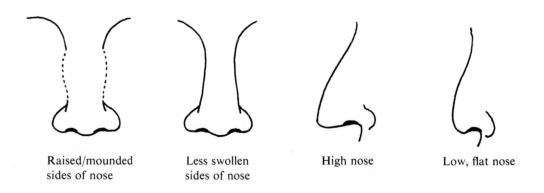

Raised/mounded
sides of nose

Less swollen
sides of nose

High nose

Low, flat nose

C. *The nostrils.* Well-developed nostrils show more determination and courage, as well as a strong masculine character, while less developed nostrils show sensitivity, gentleness, and cowardice, as well as a more feminine character (Fig. 57). In the modern age, nostrils are changing from the well-developed type to the less-developed type. Abnormally developed nostrils often demonstrate a violent character, and in the case of woman, a tendency toward lesbianism. Abnormally under-developed nostrils, in the case of man, show a lack of male vitality, and often a tendency toward homosexuality.

Fig. 57 Types of Nostrils

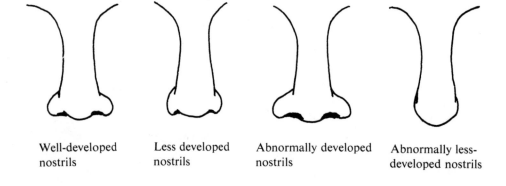

Well-developed
nostrils

Less developed
nostrils

Abnormally developed
nostrils

Abnormally less-
developed nostrils

D. *Height of the nose.* An extremely high and long nose, in the case of woman, shows an inability to conceive, and a tendency toward frigidity; while an extremely short and flat nose, in the case of man, shows low intelligence and a tendency toward physical violence (Fig. 58). In general, a high nose shows a tendency to be proud, competitive, prejudiced, and discriminating, while a lower or flatter nose indicates a tendency to be more generous and accepting of differences.

Fig. 58   Forms of the Nose (3)

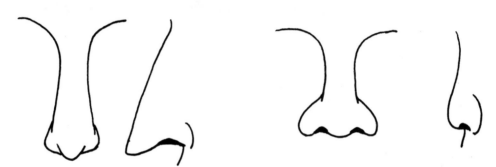

Extremely high and long nose   Extremely short and flat nose

E. *The tip of the nose.* If the end of the nose hangs down so that you cannot see both nostrils from the front, it shows a tendency toward nervousness, sensitivity and a changeable mind (Fig. 59). On the other hand, if the nose is shaped so that the two nostrils can be clearly seen from the front, narrower, unstable thinking and a more wild character are often indicated.

Fig. 59   Forms of the Nose (4)

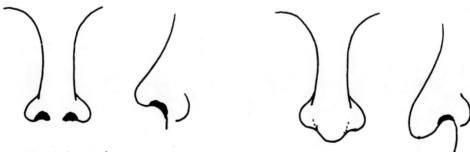

Two holes can be seen

Nose hanging down

Fig. 60 Various Forms of the Nose

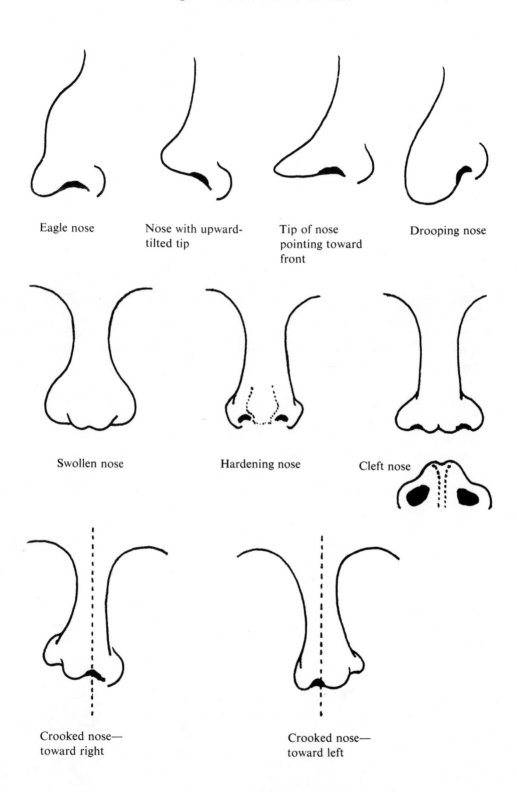

Eagle nose

Nose with upward-tilted tip

Tip of nose pointing toward front

Drooping nose

Swollen nose

Hardening nose

Cleft nose

Crooked nose—toward right

Crooked nose—toward left

2. Shape of the nose

In addition to the indications mentioned above, the specific shape of the nose indicates the specific physical and mental condition (see Fig. 60). For example:

A.   *A high, rounded shape* sometimes called an "eagle nose" is caused by the consumption of much poultry, including eggs, resulting in a tendency to be aggressive, self-centered and restless.

B.   *An upward-tilted tip of the nose* is caused by an excessive intake of animal food, especially fish and seafood, during the time of pregnancy, resulting in a tendency toward sharpness in thinking, but also in narrowness and shortsightedness.

C.   *A pointed nose*, with a tip pointing toward the front like Pinnocchio's, is caused by the overconsumption of certain kinds of fruit including melons and berries, resulting in weakness of the heart and an exciteable nervous condition.

D.   *A drooping nose* is caused by an excessive consumption of fruits and salad, as well as liquid, resulting in weakness of the heart, kidneys and bladder functions.

E.   *A swollen nose*, caused by the excessive intake of sugar, fluid, fruits, and some vegetables of tropical origin, as well as excess fats and oils, indicates that both the circulatory and excretory systems are in disorder.

F.   *A nose hardening at the tip* is caused by the intake of saturated fat, especially from animal food such as meat, poultry, eggs, cheese and other dairy products, resulting in a hardening of the arteries and muscles, and the accumulation of fat around the heart and other major compacted organs including the liver, kidneys, spleen, and prostate glands. Together with the swollen condition described above (E), this hardening nose is a sign that a heart attack or stroke may occur.

G.   *A cleft nose.*   If the tip of the nose is split or has an indentation, it is caused by nutritional imbalance, especially a shortage of minerals and complex sugars during the time of pregnancy. This condition can also be produced by an excessive intake of simple sugars such as fruits, juices, and refined sugar, as well as soft drinks, all of which deprive the body of minerals and complex sugars. A cleft nose indicates that the heart is beating irregularly or murmuring. Modern people with this type of nose are becoming more and more numerous.

H. *A crooked nose* results when the physical and mental constitutions of the parents are imbalanced, and shows an inharmonious character and physical condition.

> —*A nose bending toward the left* shows that the left side of the body —including the left lung, the spleen and pancreas, left kidney, descending colon, left ovary or testicle—are more active than the organs on the right side. This constitution shows that the father's hereditary factors were stronger.
> —*A nose bending toward the right* shows that the organs on the right of the body—including the right lung, the liver, gallbladder, right kidney, ascending colon, right ovary or testicle—are more active than the organs on the left side. In this case, the mother's hereditary factors were superior.

3.   The color of the nose

A.   A red color on the tip of the nose, resulting from the expansion of blood capillaries, is due to an excessive intake of liquid, alcohol, stimulant and aromatic beverages and seasonings, as well as fruits, juices and sugar. This condition often shows an abnormal condition of the heart, especially irregularity of blood pressure, toward hypertension.

B.   A purple nose, which is a more extreme case of the above-described red condition, often shows low blood pressure (hypotension), leading toward heart failure.

C.   Expanded capillaries appearing on the surface skin of the nose also indicate a dangerous heart and circulatory condition, as in the case of a purple nose.

D.   White nose.   When the color of the nose becomes whitish, it demonstrates a possible contraction of the heart and blood capillaries, due to an overconsumption of salt or a lack of fresh vegetables and liquid. This condition shows a timid and hesitating mentality, and physically, coldness in the peripheral areas of the body, including the fingers, toes, and general skin surface of the whole body.

4.   Pimples and patches on the nose

A.   Yellow-white pimples or patches appearing on any part of the nose show the discharge of excessive animal fat, especially dairy products. In this case, the digestive and excretory functions are in disorder.

B. Red or dark spots appearing on any part of the nose show the discharge of excessive sugar, including refined sugar, honey and fruit sugar. In this case, the excretory and circulatory functions are in disorder.

The Cheeks

Fig. 61   The Cheeks

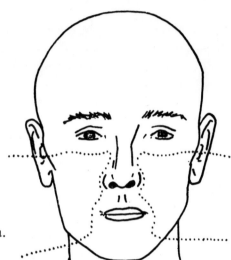

The cheek area represents the respiratory and circulatory systems, and the peripheral part of this area represents the digestive system (Fig. 61).

1.   The condition of the skin and flesh on the cheeks

A.   Cheeks with well-developed, firm flesh and a clean, clear skin color show sound respiratory and digestive functions, especially if there are no wrinkles or pimples in this area.

B.   Cheek flesh that is thinner than normal shows a lack of balanced nutrition, and especially a lack of protein and fat. Respiratory and digestive capacities are less than normal.

C.   Tight flesh on the cheeks, however, does not show an underdeveloped condition, but rather, shows active and sound functions in the above-mentioned systems.

2.   Colors and marks on the cheeks

The color of the cheeks, marks on the cheeks, and the skin condition reflect very clearly the internal conditions of the respiratory, circulatory, and digestive systems. Guidelines are as follows:

A.   Clean, clear color without pimples and wrinkles shows good health.

B.   Red or pink cheeks, except during vigorous exercise or when out in cold weather, show abnormal expansion of the blood capillaries, caused by heart and circulatory disorders due to the overconsumption of yin foods and drinks, including liquid, fruits, juices, sugars and drugs. In this case, there is a tendency toward hypertension, and mentally, a nervous sensitivity. Breathing is also faster than normal, and the speed of blood circulation is relatively fast.

C.   Milky white cheeks are caused by the overconsumption of dairy products, such as cheese, milk, cream, and yoghurt, and the overconsumption of tofu or other soybean products. An excessive intake of flour products and fruits also produces a similar color, a pinkish shade mixed with the milky white color. This condition manifests the accumulation of mucus and fat in various regions of the body, including the lungs, intestines, and reproductive organs.

D.   *Dark spots on the cheeks* are a sign of fat or mucus accumulation in some part of the lungs, often the beginning of cyst or tumor formation. Coffee and other stimulant, aromatic beverages contribute to the appearance of this color on the cheeks.

E.   *Pimples* on the cheeks show the elimination of excessive fat and mucus caused by the intake of animal food, dairy products, and oils and fats. In this case, a heavy accumulation of fat and mucus is proceeding in the lungs, intestines, reproductive organs as well as in the forebrain region. A vaginal discharge or cyst formation may be developing. If these pimples are whitish in color, the main cause is milk and sugar; while if they are yellowish, the main cause is cheese, poultry and eggs. Pimples which appear in the center of the cheeks and have a fatty appearance show the formation of cysts in the ovarian region in the case of woman, and in and around the prostate glands in the case of man.

F.   *A green shade* around the edges of the cheeks shows that cancer is proceeding either in the lungs or in the large intestine.

G.   *A dark shade* at the top of the cheekbone or the bottom of the eye region shows disorders in the kidneys and excretory system as well as in the intestines, due to the overconsumption of sugar, honey, and other sweets. This condition may also be caused by excessive salt and dried foods.

H.   *Swollen wrinkles* on the cheekbone indicate swollenness and fat or mucus accumulation in the intestinal tract, together with the overconsumption of liquid.

I.   *Freckles* on the cheeks show the elimination of simple sugars, including refined cane sugar, fruit sugar, and milk sugar, as in the case of all freckles. However, freckles on the cheeks especially indicate that these sugars are harming the respiratory and digestive functions.

J.   *A purple color*, if it appears in a large area like a shadow, indicates a serious weakening of the respiratory organs due to the overconsumption of sugar, chemicals, drugs and medicines. If it appears in small areas, it indicates blood stagnation or internal hemorrhage arising in the lungs.

K. *A pale color* shows a generally anemic condition due to imbalanced nourishment, and often it shows lung tuberculosis. In the event a pale color changes toward a more transparent shade, a tubercular condition is advancing, and leprosy and other bacterial diseases may be arising in other cases. Together with heavy animal food consumption, the intake of sugar, fruits, juices, chemicals and drugs accelerate this extremely yin, weakening condition.

L. *Grey-blue color.* This color appearing on the cheeks shows chronic liver disorders caused by the excessive intake of salt, dried foods, meat, eggs, alcohol, and sugars, both yin and yang foods. In this case, the metabolism of the liver and gallbladder is slow due to hardening or constriction in these organs.

M. *If hairs appear on the cheek*, especially fine, small, silver hairs, it indicates an overconsumption of dairy products, showing a malfunction of the reproductive organs as well as a lowered capacity in the respiratory and digestive functions.

The Ears

The ears represent the entire physical and mental constitution and condition, and especially the kidneys as their antagonstic and complementary organs. Disorders of the ears are therefore related to disorders in certain organs or glands in the body, and in particular, the kidneys and excretory functions.

Fig. 62   Forms of the Ear

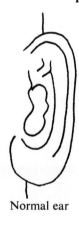

Normal ear

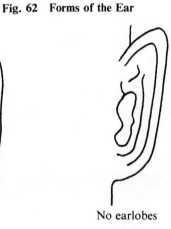

No earlobes

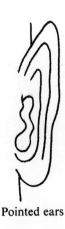

Pointed ears

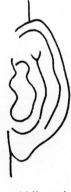

Large middle region of ear

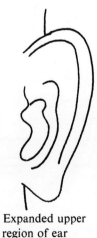

Expanded upper region of ear

1. The position and shape of the ears

The position and shape of the ears reflect the diet that was eaten by the mother during the period of pregnancy (see Fig. 62):

A. *A normal, healthy constitution* formed by balanced food during the time of pregnancy results in ears that begin at eye level and extend down to mouth level at the earlobe. The lower part of the ear should attach to the head around nose level.

B. *A small earlobe, or no earlobe*, indicates an imbalanced diet, especially lacking in minerals. This condition reflects brain and nervous functions lacking in harmonious, broad thinking.

C. *Pointed ears* result from an excessive consumption of animal protein, and show a tendency toward aggressiveness and a narrow mind and attitude.

D. *A large middle region* of the ear in proportion to the upper and lower portions indicates the overconsumption of raw vegetables and fruits, especially those of tropical origin, and a tendency to be skeptical, nervous, and often timid in thinking and attitude.

E. *Ears positioned high* on the head are caused by excessive animal food consumed during the period of pregnancy (Fig. 63). In this case, the person may be more aggressive and sharp, but lacking in well-balanced thinking and attitude.

Fig. 63   Position of the Ears

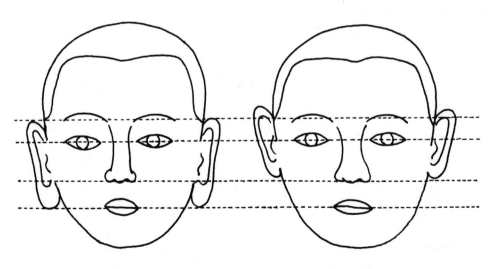

Normal position   High position

F.   Small ears are caused by the overconsumption of animal food, especially meat, poultry and eggs, and the overconsumption of baked flour products during the pregnancy period. A person with small ears tends to think of more immediate problems and with a more conceptual orientation, but is unable to think with a broad mind and understanding of the surroundings. The bigger the ears, the better the constitution.

G.   Thick ears are a sign of richness in life experience, and are caused by well-balanced nutritional factors, resulting in a sound mental and physical condition.

H.   Thin ears result from a lack of proper nutritional balance, and show a tendency toward discrimination and prejudice, with a potential for poverty and difficulties in physical and mental life.

I.   Ears lying flat close to the head, to the extent that they seem almost attached to the head, are the result of sound, balanced, well-cooked food before and after birth. They show physical and mental soundness with harmonius metabolism, and the potential to be a good social leader.

J.   Ears slightly separated from the head, within about a 30 degrees' angle of the head, are caused by the consumption of more yin foods, including leafy and raw vegetables, fruits and juices, and show a tendency to develop more mental activity than physical activity.

K.   Ears that stick out beyond a 30-degree angle are caused by the over-consumption of more extremely yin foods, including sugar, fruits, juices, chemicals and drugs, and show a tendency toward skepticism, suspicion, discrimination and narrowness in daily behavior (Fig. 64).

Fig. 64   Angle of the Ears

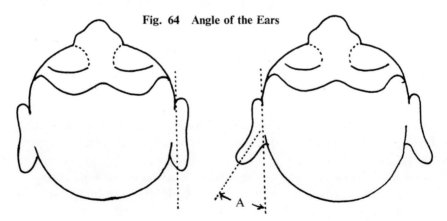

Normal ears lie flat against
the head.

If Angle A is more than 30
degrees, it is abnormal.

Fig. 65   Areas of the Ears

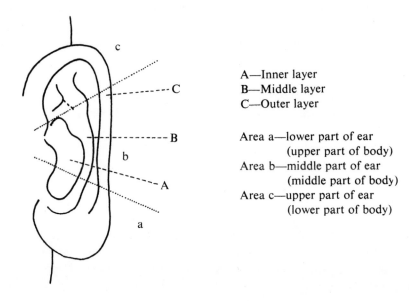

A—Inner layer
B—Middle layer
C—Outer layer

Area a—lower part of ear
         (upper part of body)
Area b—middle part of ear
         (middle part of body)
Area c—upper part of ear
         (lower part of body)

2.   The three layers of the ear

The three layers of the ear, like the three major lines on the palm, correspond with the fundamental systems in the embryonic structure during the evolutionary process of the pregnancy period (Fig. 65):

    Inner layer ....Digestive and respiratory systems
    Middle layer ....Nervous system
    Outer layer ....Circulatory and excretory systems

In these areas corresponding to each system, points are located that represent certain organs and glands. These points are located from the lower part of the ear toward the upper part of the ear, corresponding inversely with the regions of the body, upper regions to lower regions.

Accordingly, the region of the earlobe corresponds to the brain and face, and the upper part of the ears corresponds to the intestines, bladder, reproductive organs, and lower spine.

Each layer of the ear, as well as the specific location in the layer, thus represents certain organs and functions of the body. By examining a certain place on the ear, we can see the internal condition of a certain part of the body. This principle is used in acupuncture, massage treatment, and other therapies, using approximately 200 points on the ear.

A.   The small flap of cartilage at the front center of the ear.   If this flap is well-developed and protrudes more than usual, it shows strong will, tolerance, perseverance, and resistance in the physical and mental constitution.

B.   The inner layer of the ear (area A in Fig. 65) represents the digestive and respiratory regions. If it has an abnormal color or expanded blood capillaries, it shows digestive and respiratory disorders.

C.   The middle layer (area B) represents the nervous system. If it protrudes abnormally, it shows a nature that is persistent, self-imposing and stubborn. A red color in this area shows nervous disorders.

D.   The outer layer (area C) shows the circulatory and excretory system. If it has an abnormally red color, except during vigorous exercise or outdoors in cold weather, it indicates spleen and lymphatic disorders.

E.   A purple color shows weak circulatory functions due to consumption of extremely yin foods and drinks.

F.   The upper area of the ear (area c), if it is enlarged abnormally, shows a potential for development of hyper- or hypo-glycemia, due to an overconsumption of sugar, fruits and dairy products during the time of pregnancy.

G.   If the earlobe is clearly separated from the head, and is well-developed, it is an indication of clear brain and nervous functions and, in the case of woman, sound reproductive organs.

4. The Forehead

The forehead reflects the entire physical and mental constitution, and each area of the forehead corresponds to certain areas of the body. Everyone's forehead is different, and conditions of its shape, color, skin, and other characteristics reveal physical and mental constitutional and conditional variations. The forehead can be divided into four areas (Fig. 66): the lower forehead (A), the middle forehead (B), the upper forehead (C), and the temples (D).

1.   The lower forehead

This area represents, physically, the digestive and respiratory systems and and their functions; and psychologically, sensory discrimination and practicality. If the bone and muscle structure develops well in this area, it shows

Fig. 66 Areas of the Forehead Corresponding to Areas of the Body

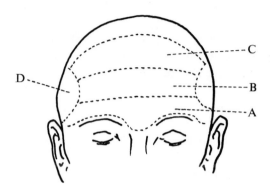

A. Lower region—Digestive and respiratory systems
B. Middle region—Nervous system
C. Upper region—Circulatory and excretory systems
D. Temples region—Spleen, pancreas, liver and gallbladder

that these digestive and respiratory functions are strong and sound, and physcial and mental energies are active in daily practical life. A change of color and other abnormal symptoms in this region indicate a change of internal conditions. For example:

A. *A red color* shows that the digestive functions are disordered, with expansion of parts of the digestive vessel such as the stomach and intestines, due to an overconsumption of animal fat, vegetable oil, fruits, juices, sugar, alcohol, and liquid, as well as other very yin foods and drinks. It is also a sign that inflammation may be developing in the respiratory or digestive organs, with an accumulation of fat and mucus in both the lungs and large intestines.

B. *A dark color* indicates slow metabolism in the respiratory and digestive functions, mainly due to an overconsumption of yang foods such as meat, eggs, salts, dried foods, baked flour products, and others. Constipation and breathing difficulties may be present.

C. *A green color* shows an accumulation of mucus and fat developing toward the formation of cysts, tumors and cancer in the respiratory or digestive systems, due to an overconsumption of animal fat, dairy food, and yin foods and drinks such as fruits, juices, soft drinks, refined flour products, chemicals, drugs, and medications.

D. *White or yellow patches, pimples and spots* represent the elimination of mucus and fat accumulated in the lungs and intestines, mainly due to the overconsumption of poultry, eggs, cheese, milk, and other dairy products.

E. *Red pimples* show an elimination of excessively yin foods, including fruits, juices, sugars, chemicals and others.

F. *The central region of the lower forehead* represents the condition of the liver and gallbladder (Fig. 67). For example:

Fig. 67   The Forehead–Central Region

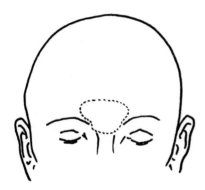 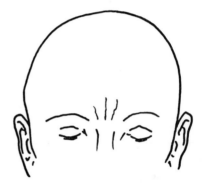

Central region of the lower part
of the forehead

Signs of liver disorder

1. Vertical wrinkles appearing in this region—very common among modern people—are a sign of accumulation of mucus and fat in the liver, and expansion or hardening of the liver. The deeper and longer the wrinkles are, the worse the condition is. There may be only one wrinkle, or several. If only one or two, the liver is harder and more rigid, with stagnation in its functions. These vertical lines have been known as a sign of anger, and therefore the words for anger, *kan shaku* (肝癪), which have been used in Japan and China for centuries, are written with two characters meaning "liver pains," or acute disease of the liver. These wrinkles represent not only physical disorders in the liver and gallbladder, but also a mental tendency toward upset, short temper and excitement.

2. If this area has white or yellow patches together with vertical lines, it indicates the development of cyst or tumor formation in the liver, or stone formation in the gallbladder.

3. Pimples in this area, with or without wrinkles, show hard fat deposits in the liver, or stone formation in the gallbladder, due to a long-time consumption of animal fat, including dairy products. This also indicates mental inflexibility.

4. Dry, flaky skin in this region, possibly extending into the region above the eyebrows, shows an over consumption of fats and oils from both animal and vegetable sources, together with flour products, and a lack of adequate vegetable consumption.

2. The middle forehead

This area shows the nervous system's condition. If the area is well-developed, it indicates a sound intellectual capacity. If this area is indented in relation to the upper and lower regions of the forehead, natural instincts are active. Changes in color and other symptoms in this region show various nervous disorders. For example:

A. *A red color* shows nervousness, oversensitivity, excitability, and instability, due to the overconsumption of yin foods, including stimulants, aromatic beverages, fruits, juices, soft drinks, and others.

B. *A white color* is caused by an overconsumption of dairy products, especially milk, cream and yoghurt, together with excessive liquid. Nervous functions are generally slow and dull, and mental activities are cloudy and unclear.

C. *A yellow color* shows that nervous functions tend to be alert, but narrow and inflexible. Although the major cause is the excessive intake of eggs, poultry and dairy food, in some instances a similar condition may also be produced by the overconsumption of root vegetables, such as carrots. In either case, the underlying disorder indicated is abnormal functioning of the liver and gallbladder.

D. *Dark spots and patches*, usually called "freckles," in this area as well as in any other area of the forehead, show the elimination of excessive sugars, fruits, juices, honey, milk sugar, and other sweets, as well as chemicals, drugs and medications.

E. *Red pimples or spots* also show the elimination of similar yin foods, but emphasizing more sugar and fruits combined with refined white flour products or dairy products. However, this condition is more temporary compared to a condition of freckles or dark spots.

3. The upper forehead

The upper region of the forehead immediately below the hairline represents the circulatory and excretory systems and their functions. If this region is well-developed, it shows sound circulatory and excretory functions, including sound conditions of the heart, kidneys and bladder. However, if this region is not developed, these systems are weaker than normal. This region also represents the spiritual character, which is parallel to the degree of development of this region: if it is well-developed and well-balanced in form, it shows a sound spiritual capability, including an understanding of the invisible mental/spiritual world, with a larger view than usual.

Changes in color, hairs, and other appearances in this region indicate various physical, mental and spiritual tendencies. For example:

A. *A red color* shows that the circulatory functions are overworking due to excessive consumption of liquids, fruits, juices and other yin foods and drinks, including alcohol, stimulant and aromatic beverages. This causes a faster pulse and in some cases produces fever. The excretory functions also become overactive, with frequent urination, indigestion and diarrhea.

B. *A white color and white patches* appear due to the overconsumption of fats and oils, including dairy products as well as fats and oils from both animal and vegetable sources. This condition is often accompanied by silver "baby hairs" caused by the overconsumption of milk and other dairy products. A high cholesterol and fatty acid content may be observed in the bloodstream. Weakening heartbeat as well as accumulation of fat and mucus in the kidneys, ureter, and other excretory organs are indicated.

C. *Dark color and patches* are caused by the consumption of excess sugars, including sugars from fruits and juices, milk, and cane. Honey, syrups and refined white flour products are not excepted. The kidneys may be forming deposits of fat and mucus, cysts and stones, and bladder infections may occur easily.

D. *Yellow color and patches* show the elimination of excessive animal fat, especially from meat, poultry, eggs and cheese. Fish oils can also contribute to this condition. The bloodstream in this condition has a high cholesterol and fatty acid content, and the functions of the liver and gallbladder are in disorder.

E. *Pimples* in this area show the elimination of different types of food consumed in excess: red pimples from sugar, fruits and juices; white pimples from fats and oils; yellowish pimples from animal fats and cholesterol; and dark pimples from protein and fat together, as in the case of moles and warts.

F. *Receding hair* in this region, resulting in a bald forehead region, is caused by the overconsumption of yin foods, including liquids, alcohol, fruits, juices, sugars and other sweets (see p. 104). It shows that the heart and circulatory functions are overworking due to a larger volume of blood and lymph fluid, and a thinner quality of these fluids. The excretory functions are overactive, and especially urination is overactive and frequent.

4. The temples

The temples correspond to the functions of the spleen, pancreas, liver and gallbladder. For example:

A. *Green vessels* appearing in this region show abnormal lymph circulation due to an overactive spleen or underactive gallbladder, and are caused by excess fluid and sugar, fats and oils, alcohol and stimulants, and other yin foods and drinks.

B. *A dark color* shows the elimination of excess sugars including cane sugar, honey, syrups, chocolate, fruits, juices and milk. This condition also arises sometimes from the opposite cause—excess consumption of salts and salt-treated foods, as well as dried foods. This condition shows that the liver, spleen and kidneys are underactive. The pancreatic functions also tend to produce an irregular sugar level, resulting in such conditions as hyperglycemia and hypoglycemia.

C. *Patches and pimples* appearing in this region also show the elimination of various excesses from dairy products. Red pimples and patches are caused by excess sugar, sweets, fruits and juices. Whitish yellow pimples are caused by fats and oils from both animal and vegetable sources. Dark patches and pimples are caused by excessive sweets, or else by salt and flour products. Moles and warts are caused by excess proteins and fat together. These show, respectively, disorders in the spleen and pancreas, liver and gallbladder.

5. The forehead as a whole

The entire forehead shows the entire physical condition, and the nervous system in particular.

A. *A forehead that is clean and clear* with normal skin conditions shows physical and mental health, with all metabolisms in harmony.

B. *A watery forehead*, especially the upper region, shows disorders in the circulatory and excretory systems due to excessive liquid consumption, including fruits and fruit juices.

C. *An oily skin condition* indicates disorders in the liver, the gallbladder, and the digestive system, due to an overconsumption of oily foods, including fats and oils from both animal and vegetable sources.

D. *Horizontal wrinkles* on the forehead, which arise early in adulthood, are caused by excess liquid including all beverages, fruits, fruit juice and dairy products, often together with excess fats and oils (Fig. 68). However, horizontal wrinkles appearing on the forehead after the age of 50 are more natural, due to the construction of the tissues of the forehead. These lines represent the major systems of the body, as follows. If four lines appear, do not count either the top or the bottom line, whichever one is weaker; and if five lines appear, discount the top and bottom lines.

Fig. 68   Horizontal Wrinkles on the Forehead

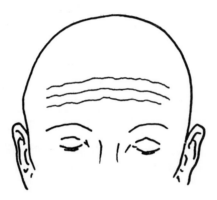

—*Bottom lines:*   The digestive and respiratory systems, corresponding to the life line on the palm.
—*Middle line:*   The nervous system, corresponding to the line of intellect on the palm.
—*The upper line:*   The circulatory and excretory systems, corresponding to the line of emotion on the palm.

These three lines should be long, deep and clear in the case of a healthy physical and mental condition. If any of them is weak, dim and broken, that particular system is weak. If red, dark, white or yellow spots appear on any line, it indicates a certain disordered area in that system.

E. *Hairs growing on the forehead* show the overconsumption of certain foods:

—*White, silvery hairs* are caused by dairy products.
—*Dark brown hairs* are caused by carbohydrates.
—*Fine, brown-yellow hairs* are caused by animal protein and fat.

5. The Hair

Hair growing on any part of the body is the elimination of excessive nourishment. The main substance of the hair is protein, fat and minerals, but they are also produced by the consumption of carbohydrates, which turn into protein and fat in the body. Hair can be divided into two general categories:

1. Hair that grows in an upward direction, such as head hair.
2. Hair that grows in a downward direction, such as the moustache, beard, and most body hair.

Upward-growing hair results more from vegetable quality foods, including carbohydrates, while downward-growing hair results more from protein and fat from both animal and vegetable sources.

Hair resembles growing trees and plants on the surface of the earth. The quality of the hair—its hardness or softness, lightness or darkness, wetness or dryness, its length, and other characteristics—clearly show our physical and mental constitutions and conditions. For example, people who live in a northern climate with less sunshine usually have blonde or brown hair with a fine, soft texture; and people who live in a warmer climate with strong sunshine produce darker and harder hair. These climatic differences result in differences in diet, producing different kinds of hair, according to the following principles:

Climate	Dietary Practive	Type of Hair
Cold (yin)	More animal food, dairy products, fish, and seasonal, well-cooked grains and vegetables; more salt (yang).	Blonde, red, brunette; fine, thin, softer, and curved hair (yin).
Cool, four-season climate (yin)	Well-cooked grains and vegetables, with occasional fruits. Animal food, dairy products, fish and seafood (yang).	Brunette, brown and black; soft but slightly harder. Straighter, less curved (yin).
Warmer four-season climate (yang)	Grains, vegetables and fruits, including raw vegetables and fruits, with little animal food, dairy products, fish or seafood (yin).	Dark or black; harder and straight (yang).

Climate	Dietary Practice	Type of Hair
Hot semi-tropical climate (yang)	Grains, vegetables, including raw foods, fresh fruits and juices; very little animal food, dairy food, fish or seafood (yin).	Black, hard and curly (yang).

According to these principles, a yang physical condition, nourished by yang foods, produces a yin type of hair; and a yin physical condition, nourished by yin foods, produces a yang type of hair. It is thus easy to understand why an infant, who has a more yang condition (smaller size, higher temperature, etc.) produces a yin type of hair—soft and curving with a lighter color—and as it grows, the hair changes to become harder and straighter with a darker color, generally speaking.

Hair appears on various parts of the body, and by examining its color, texture and other characteristics, we can diagnose the conditions of the various organs and functions that correspond to its specific appearance, as discussed below.

1. Hair on the head

The hair on the head is a good reflection of our physical and mental condition, and especially shows our condition during the time the hair was growing. Each strand of hair represents all phases of the entire growing period, the end of the strand reflecting the past, and the root area reflecting the present. A microscopic examination would show distinct variations in thickness, color, hardness, texture and curliness along one strand of hair (Fig. 69). If we examine a strand of hair that has taken one year to grow, we can divide it into sections representing the four seasons or the twelve

Fig. 69 A Strand of Head Hair, Showing Past and Recent Growth Patterns

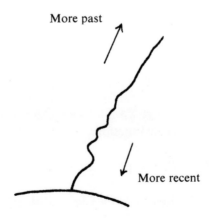

More past

More recent

months. The condition of each section reveals what kinds of food and drink were consumed, what types of sickness were experienced, and what mental states were occurring. The following are general guidelines:

Hair Quality	Type of Nourishment
Thicker; lighter	More protein and fat
Thicker; darker	More carbohydrates, vegetable protein and oils
Thinner; lighter	More animal-quality foods, or well-cooked vegetables foods with salt.
Thinner; darker	More well-cooked vegetable-quality foods with salt.
Curly	More animal-quality foods with salt, under temperate climatic conditions; more carbo-hydrates with strong sunshine under tropical climatic conditions.
Straight	Both vegetable and animal foods; generally well-balanced.
Grey or white	More animal foods or well-cooked vegetables with salt; sometimes, malnutrition.

However, it should be remembered that hair grows more slowly in the late fall and winter, and faster in the spring and summer, so that the seasonal sections of hair will not be of equal length.

The hair on the head can be divided into several areas which correspond with certain regions of the body (Fig. 70):

Hair Region	Region of Body
Front (A)	Kidney, bladder, the excretory system and its functions.
Side (B)	Lungs, large intestines and their functions.
Top (C)	Heart, circulatory system, small intestines and their functions.
Side near the back (D)	Spleen-pancreas, stomach and their functions.
Back (E)	Liver, gallbladder and their functions

Fig. 70   Head Hair and Related Parts of Body

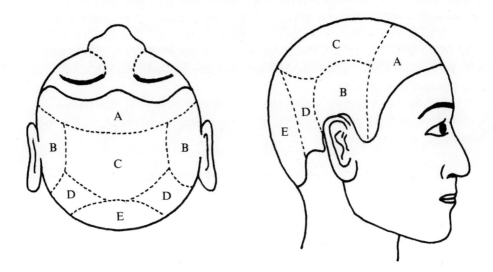

Hair also shows the inner and peripheral conditions of the body: the ends of the hair show the more inner regions of the body, and the roots, the more peripheral regions.

Accordingly, changes in color and other characteristics arising in certain areas of the head indicate the condition of the corresponding systems, organs, glands and functions of the body.

A.   Split ends are a manifestation of a yin condition of differentiation or branching out, and indicate that the inner region of the body is affected by an overconsumption of yin foods—overeating in general, including sugar and sweets, oils and fats, fruits and juices, and a lack of hard, fibrous grains, vegetables and seaweed as well as properly balanced minerals (Fig. 71). This condition especially reveals that the ovaries and uterus, prostate gland and testicles, and the reproductive functions in general are not in sound condition.

Fig. 71   Split Ends of Hair

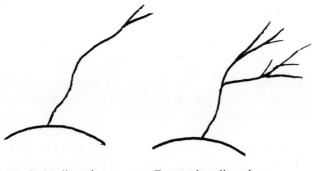

Typical split ends   Extremely split ends

B. Grey and white hair develops naturally with age. This is a good example to demonstrate that an excessively yang, contracting physical condition produces this color. If excess animal food or well-cooked vegetable foods are eaten, with a relatively large volume of salt and minerals, and without sufficient fresh, leafy vegetables, this color can easily occur. The consumption of grey sea salt, or baked and roasted flour products treated with salt, can also produce this condition.

As the hair turns grey or white, the liver and gallbladder functions become underactive, and the personality becomes more determined, rigid, and stubborn, with a narrow mind.

C. Wet and dry hair. The consumption of liquid, including all beverages, fruits, fruit juices and other liquid used in cooking, produce more wet hair. In this case, the circulatory and excretory functions are overactive, with overactive and frequent urination.

On the other hand, dehydration results in dry hair. In this case, in addition to liver and gallbladder functions, the functions of the spleen and pancreas are also abnormal, with stagnation in the circulatory and respiratory functions.

D. Oily hair. Overconsumption of fat and oil from both animal and vegetable sources, but not to the extent that fat accumulation underneath the skin prevents perspiration, produces oily hair. The fats and oils that cause this type of hair are more of the unsaturated kind.

In this case, mucus accumulation may be proceeding in the lungs, intestines, and reproductive organs due to the increased fatty acid content of the bloodstream, resulting in underactivity of the respiratory, digestive and reproductive functions, and producing general fatigue and laziness.

E. Dandruff is an elimination of excessive food, especially proteins and fats, that results in peeling skin. It can be caused by overeating in general; or by the overconsumption of any kind of animal food; or by oily and fatty foods of both animal and vegetable quality. Dandruff indicates, physically, disorders in the kidneys and excretory functions; and psychologically, a changeable mind, indecisiveness, excitability and a short temper.

2. Hair loss

Hair loss is common among modern people. It can occur in patches, or in one of three general types of baldness. All hair loss results from one of two major causes, as discussed below:

A. Hair loss at the front sides of the head is due to the expansion of tissues, caused by the overconsumption of liquid and other yin foods and

Fig. 72 Areas of Hair Loss

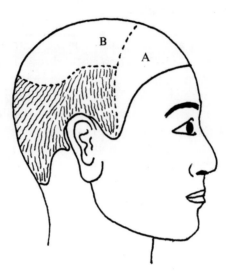

drinks, including all beverages, fruits, juices, soft drinks, sugars, sweets, stimulants, chemicals, drugs, medications, raw vegetables, tomatoes, eggplant and other vegetables of tropical origin (Area A in Fig. 72).

In this condition, the heart and circulatory functions, kidneys and excretory functions, and the reproductive vitalities are declining. The digestive functions, especially intestinal activities, may also be underactive. Mentally, there is a tendency to be more conceptual and intellectual, rather than practical and materialistic.

B. Hair loss in the central region of the head arises when there is an overconsumption of yang foods, including meat, poultry, eggs, dairy food, and in some cases, fish and seafood (Area B in Fig. 72). Animal protein, heavy saturated fats, salt, and dry foods cause this type of baldness.

In this case, the heart, liver, pancreas and reproductive organs are gathering an accumulation of fat and mucus, resulting in hardness and rigidity in the muscles and tissues. This condition tends to produce cardiovascular disorders, chronic digestive trouble, and the formation of cysts and tumors. Mentally, it shows a more aggressive, offensive and determined attitude, with an orientation toward practical and materialistic thinking.

C. Hair loss in the front and central regions of the head, covering a large area, is caused by a combination of the two conditions described above (items A and B): both extremes of heavy yang animal food and yin foods such as sugar, fruits, juices, chemicals and drugs, and a lack of balanced nutritional factors from grains, beans, vegetables and seaweed.

Therefore, a variety of physical symptoms arise, including acute and degenerative diseases. Mentally, there is a tendency to develop a schizophrenic condition, changes of mood, irritability, with a lack of steadiness, patience, generosity, compassion and perseverance.

D. Hair loss in patches may arise temporarily in a certain area of the head, due to one or two types of food, as described above. The location of this kind of hair loss indicates a temporary disorder in the corresponding region of the body. For example, hair loss in patches at the top of the head near the hair spiral is due to a sudden overconsumption of animal food, disturbing the functions of the small intestine. If the hair loss occurs at the sides of the head, it is caused by a sudden intake of a large amount of animal fats, dairy products, and vegetable oils, with fruits or fruit juices, which is temporarily disturbing the functions of the lungs.

Especially if these patches are accompanied by flaking skin, a discharge of animal-quality fats is indicated.

3. Moustaches and beards

Moustaches and beards are also eliminations of excessive food, and like head hair, are normal processes of discharge. They normally appear in men and not in women. If a man does not have a moustache and beard, it is an abnormal condition, as when a woman has a moustache and beard. Since the area around the mouth corresponds to the genital area, the moustache and beard are closely connected with the condition and function of the male and female hormones.

General guidelines for diagnosis are as follows:

A. A heavier moustache and beard indicates more nourishment, including overeating and a faster metabolism. The overconsumption of animal-quality foods creates a much heavier moustache and beard than vegetable-quality foods, although vegetable foods can also produce them actively if eaten to excess. This condition shows a more physical nature, with a tendency to be strong but mentally rough.

B. A thinner moustache and beard indicates less nourishment, especially less protein and fat, and slower metabolism. Since the speed of growth of the moustache and beard is proportional to metabolic activity, a person who is less physically active has a more slowly-growing moustache and beard. In this case, there is a tendency to have a more mental, esthetic and delicate nature.

C. A moustache or beard appearing on a woman is caused by a diet rich in animal-quality foods, or protein and fat, or by overeating in general. Women should have no moustache or beard, and when they appear, it indicates disorders in the reproductive functions.

D. A moustache and beard covering an unusually large area, especially on the cheek region, is caused by an overconsumption of dairy products or other animal fats. In this case, the reproductive activity is lower than average, and mental capacities are rather limited, especially the capacity for higher spiritual functions.

4. Hair on the body

Hair appears on many areas of the body, and it is different in every person, according to variations in diet followed since the time of pregnancy. In general, we can see a few basic patterns relating to hair growth:

—Asian races have less body hair than occidental races.
—People living in hot or warmer climates have less body hair than people living in colder climates.
—People who have eaten vegetable-quality foods have less body hair than people who have eaten animal-quality foods.
—Women have less body hair than men.

The amount of body hair tends to decrease as biological evolution progresses toward higher species. The shells of invertebrates and amphibians, the scales of fish and reptiles, have evolved into body hair in mammals. As mammals develop toward the human state, body hair rapidly disappears, and

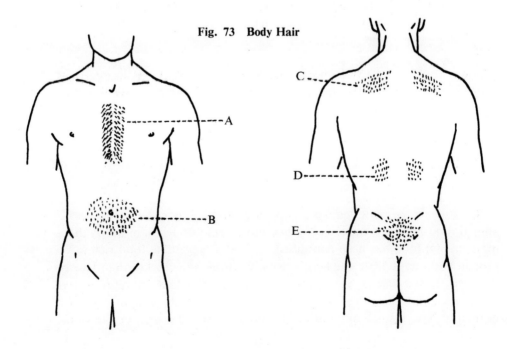

Fig. 73   Body Hair

is completely absent in woman—the highest stage of biological evolution on earth at present.

Those who have body hair, therefore, whether men or women, have not been following a daily diet suitable for human beings—cereal grains and vegetables—but have been eating other types of food, including meat, poultry, eggs, dairy products, sugar, and food rich in protein and fat of both animal and vegetable quality.

A. Diagnosis of body hair. Depending on its location, body hair shows different causes and conditions, as follows (see Fig. 73):

Location	Cause	Condition
Chest region (A)	Animal fat, dairy products, vegetable oil.	Weakness in bronchi, lungs, and respiratory functions.
Abdominal region (B)	Animal protein, saturated fats.	Weakness in intestines and digestive functions.
Upper back region (C)	Both animal and vegetable fats; overconsumption of sugar and other carbohydrates.	Weakness in lungs and respiratory functions.
Middle back region (D)	Excess dairy products and other animal fats; vegetables fats; overconcumption of protein.	Weakness in kidneys and excretory functions.
Lower back region (E)	Excess animal and vegetable food rich in protein and fat.	Weakness in intestines and digestive functions.
Hair in any place	Excess animal and vegetable protein and fat.	Weakness in the organ and its function located in that place.

B. Hair on the arms and legs. Less arm and leg hair shows that less animal food has been consumed, while more arm and leg hair shows that more animal food has been consumed, as well as vegetable food rich in protein and fat. Hair on the legs is usually harder and thicker than hair on the arms. In the case of woman, thick leg hairs show that the reproductive functions tend to be either overactive or inhibited. In the case of man, it is normal to have a small amount of hair on the arms and legs, unlike women, who have very little or none if in good health.

Arm hair of white-silver color—"baby hair"—is caused by the over-consumption of dairy products, especially milk. In this case, the respiratory and digestive functions tend to be weak, and there may be an accumulation of fat and mucus in various parts of the body.

C.   Underarm hair.   Thick, long underarm hair is caused by the over-consumption of food, and especially proteins and fats, together with excessive liquid, including all beverages, fruits and juices. In this condition, the digestive functions tend to be weaker.

Thinner and shorter underarm hair is caused by less nourishment and more consumption of vegetables and fruits than food rich in carbohydrates, protein and fat. This condition reveals a potential weakness of the respiratory and circulatory functions.

D.   Pelvic hair.   Everyone has a different condition of pelvic hair, due to differences in the physical constitution developed during the time of pregnancy, as well as differences in diet from infancy to the present. Guidelines are as follows:

Type of hair	Dietary cause	Condition
Thick pelvic hair	Rich nourishment and over-eating, especially protein and fat, mainly from animal food but also from vegetable food in some cases, including beans, nuts and other oily food.	Generally sound sexual behavior and reproductive capacity.
Thin pelvic hair	Less nourishment or less eating, especially protein and fat. More vegetable consumption with dairy food in some cases.	The sexual senses are more sensitive, but reproductive capacity is less.
Wider area of pelvic hair	Excess protein and fat, with dairy products, sugar, fruits dairy products, sugar, fruits and juices.	Less orderly sexual behavior; greater susceptibility to genital disorders.
Smaller area of pelvic	Less variety of food, especially proteins and fats.	Generally sound sexual condition and reproductive capacity.

Type of hair	Dietary cause	Condition
No pelvic hair	Overconsumption of eggs, cheese, milk and blue-skinned fish, or flour products, fruits, juices, sugars and other yin foods, with a lack of grains and vegetables.	Sexually sensitive, but less vitality and reproductive capacity.

6. The Hands

The hands and feet, as the end points of the arms and legs, may be considered as extensions of the internal organs. Therefore, they reflect the constitutions and conditions of various organs. The more peripheral areas of the hands, toward the fingertips, correspond to the deeper parts of the organs (Fig. 74). The arms, hands and fingers, as well as the legs, feet and toes, are created in a spirallic pattern growing out from the internal organs, from which energy is discharged after the organs are formed, during the embryonic period. They continue to develop after birth, and act as peripheral parts of the body for the discharge of energy, vibrations, and nutritional excesses from the inner regions of the body. Thus, they can also reveal recent and present physical and mental conditions.

Fig. 74 Arms and Legs Correlating to Internal Organs

More toward A—correlating to more peripheral parts of organs
More toward B—correlating to more deeper parts of organs

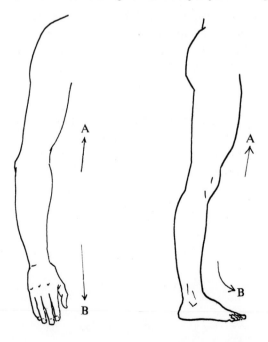

Fig. 75 Palms and Fingers Correlating to Body Functions

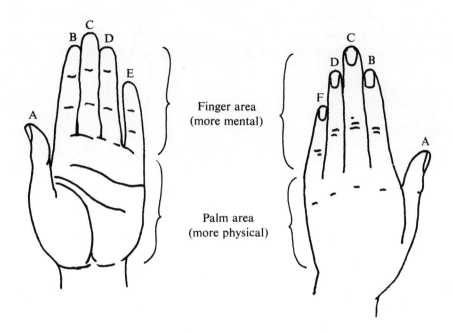

1. General characteristics of the hands

The hand can be divided into two general areas: the palm and the fingers. The palm reflects more the physical constitution, while the fingers reflect more the mental tendencies. We can also divide the hand into six regions vertically, which correlate with the six major meridians (Fig. 75):

1. The thumb and its base (A), which corresponds to the lungs and their functions.
2. The index finger and its base (B), or root, down to the base of the palm, and including the same region on the back of the hand, corresponding to the large intestine and its functions.
3. The middle finger and its root (C), including that region on the back of the hand, corresponding to the three *chakras*, which are energy centers for the heart, stomach, and abodminal regions, and the circulatory and reproductive functions.
4. The ring finger and its root (D), including the same region on the back of the hand, corresponding to the three *chakras* or energy centers in the control of vitality, temperature and energy.
5. The little finger and its root, on the palm side only (E), which corresponds to the heart and circulatory functions.
6. The little finger and its root, on the back of the hand (F), which corresponds to the small intestine and its functions.

Fig. 76   Lines on the Palm   **Fig. 77   Sections of the Fingers**

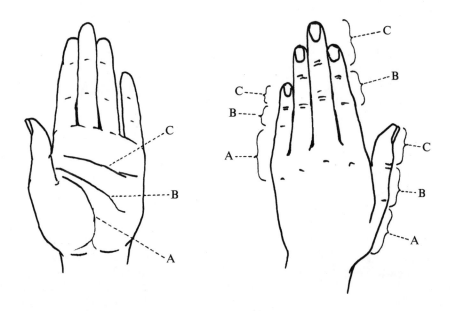

A.   The palm.   The palm can be divided into three regions following the three basic lines on the palm, which correspond to the major systems of the body (Fig. 76):

> *Line A* and its region correspond to the digestive and respiratory functions. It is called the "life line," due to its vital importance for life activity and longevity.
>
> *Line B* and its region correspond to the nervous functions. It is called the "line of intellect," since it reflects the brain and nervous qualities.
>
> *Line C* and its region correspond to the circulatory and excretory functions. It is called the "line of emotion," due to the decisive influence of the blood, lymph and urinary conditions upon emotional activity.

B.   The fingers can also be divided into three regions according to the sections marked by their knuckles (Fig. 77):

> *The base area* (A), corresponding to the digestive and respiratory functions. In the case of the thumb, this is the root region.
>
> *The middle region* (B) corresponds to the nervous functions. In the thumb, this is the base area.
>
> *The tip region* (C) corresponds to the circulatory and excretory functions.

C.   The nails are an elimination of excessive nutrients in the form of minerals and protein, as in the case of hair. They therefore represent the whole body's condition, and clearly reveal the past changing condition during the period of nail growth.

2. Special conditions of the hands, palms and fingers

Using the general guidelines described above, variations in constitution and condition can be understood as follows:

A. *Length of the palm.* If the palm is longer than the fingers, the physical constitution is well-developed, and has greater strength, resistance and perseverance. On the other hand, if the fingers are nearly the same length as the palm or, in some rare cases, longer, the mental capacities are more developed, although there is a tendency toward physical weakness.

B. *Thickness of the palm.* A thick palm represents a good constitution nourished by well-balanced foods and drinks, indicating the potential for a generally sound, healthy and prosperous life. A thin palm, caused by imbalanced nourishment, represents weaker health and vitality, with frequent struggles and hardship.

C. *Width of the palm.* A wide palm results from good, balanced food, including grains, beans, and vegetables, showing physical strength and vitality with a potentially long life. A narrow palm, on the other hand, results from the overconsumption of sugar and sweets, fruits and juices, and other yin foods, and shows a weaker constitution with a potentially short life.

D. *Wet and dry palms.* Wet palms, unpleasant during a handshake, indicate an overconsumption of liquid, including all beverages, milk, fruits, juices, sugar and sweets. The heart and circulatory functions, and the kidneys and excretory functions, are overworking due to this over-liquid condition. General fatigue, both physical and mental, is occurring. Excessive sweat and unpleasant body odors may be present. Insomnia, emotional disturbance, forgetfulness, and cloudy thinking often accompany this condition.

However, hands that are too dry indicate dehydration, and the temperature of the palms is usually cold because of the contraction of tissues, blood vessels and capillaries. The overconsumption of dried foods, animal food, salts, with a lack of fluid produces this condition. Physically and mentally, it indicates rigidity and inflexibility. Although the thinking may be sharp, there is often a tendency toward narrowness, prejudice, misunderstanding, and fanaticism. This condtion can be seen sometimes even among grain-and-vegetable eaters if they consume too much salt and too little liquid.

A normal, healthy condition will include a palm that is slightly moist with a cool temperature. The degree of moisture is very subtle, and it is almost not detectable. In this condition, the palm has a clean, clear color, and the physical metabolism and mental activities are well-coordinated. Urination is taking place three to four times per day, a healthy average for an adult.

E. The color of the palm should be clean and clear and uniform. If the periphery of the palm develops a red color, it shows that the heart and circulatory functions are overactive due to the overconsumption of stimulant beverages, fruits and juices, and other yin foods and drinks. If a purple color develops, especially in the area between the little finger and the base of the palm, it indicates disorders of the circulatory and excretory functions. If a green color arises in that area, tumors and cancer may be growing in the intestinal region.

If the palm becomes more yellow than usual, there is excessive bile secretion due to liver, gallbladder, circulatory and excretory disorders, caused by the overconsumption of animal food, including eggs, dairy food, oils and fats, and salt. This condition may be caused in some cases by an overconsumption of some root vegetables such as carrots, or some round vegetables such as pumpkin or autumn squash.

F. The color of the back of the hand may change to red or purple depending upon the environmental temperature. However, if these colors arise under normal circumstances, it indicates disorders in the circulatory, excretory, digestive and nervous systems due to imbalanced dietary habits, especially the overconsumption of yin foods as well as chemicals, drugs and medications.

If marijuana, hashish, LSD and other hallucinatory drugs, as well as medications, are used repeatedly for some period, their discharging process changes the color of the hand and fingers to red or purple, especially on the back of the hand. The time needed to eliminate these drugs and chemicals from the body can be estimated as follows:

Area where red or purple color appears	*Time needed for elimination*
Tip of fingers	Six months
Tip and middle sections of fingers	One year
The entire length of the fingers	Two years
The entire hand, including the back of the hand to the wrist	Fours years

While this elimination is proceeding, the physical metabolism and organ functions are slower than normal, especially the functions of the heart, kidneys and reproductive organs. At the same time, the brain and nervous functions remain abnormal, often showing oversensitivity, fanaticism, conceptuality, depression, excitability, instability, frustration, inner anger, cowardice, timidity, and frequent changes of mind, as well as undependability.

This physical and mental condition arises to a lesser degree if sugar and sweets, fruits and juices, dairy products and refined flour products, vitamins and supplements, and other yin foods and drinks are consumed in excess.

Fig. 78   The Root of the Thumb

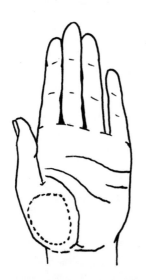

G. Change of color at the root of the thumb. If a red, blue or purple color develops at the root of the thumb between the thumb and line A, it shows that the digestive functions are in disorder, especially in the small and large intestines, due to dietary imbalance (Fig. 78). If a similar color appears on the back of the hand between the root of the thumb and the index finger, it is also an indication of digestive disorders, especially in the large intestine. A green color in that region shows the development of tumors or cancer in the colon: in the descending colon if on the left hand, and in the ascending colon if on the right hand.

H. Strength and flexibility of the hands. Thick, strong fingers with a well-developed bone structure show a strong physical constitution, especially in the nervous system. Thin, long fingers indicate a more mental and spiritual nature, with an artistic orientation. Many musicians have this type of fingers.

Flexibility of the joints of the hands and fingers shows physical and mental flexibility, while their inflexibility shows physical and mental rigidity. When the hand is fully stretched, if the fingers can curve backward, it indicates a greater mental and spiritual capacity (Fig. 79). On the other hand, if the fingers tend to curve forward when the hand is stretched, it shows mental rigidity and physical strength.

Flexibility of the joints of the fingers, hands, and wrists is important in maintaining an adaptable life. The greater the flexibility, the more capacity there is to adapt the physical and mental conditions to the environment. Loss of flexibility is due to hardening of the muscles, arteries and nervous systems, caused by an overconsumption of animal food, especially rich in protein, saturated fats and cholesterol. This condition is also accelerated by overeating in general, and by an excessive intake of salt and minerals.

Fig. 79   Test of Flexibility of the Hands

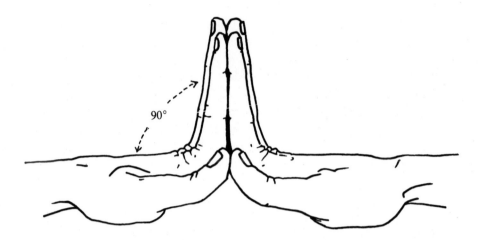

Hold the hands together; then, with the four fingers of the hands still tightly attached, bend the hands up to 90 degrees. If this cannot be done, it indicates inflexibility and the potential for hardening of the arteries, nerves, and muscles

Fig. 80   Webbed Fingers

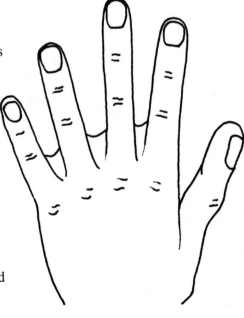

I.   Webbed fingers.   When the fingers are spread, tiny webs appear between them at their roots (Fig. 80). If these webs are abnormally large, it indicates that more yin foods were eaten by the mother during the early part of pregnancy, including chemicals, drugs and medications. If the webs are small, an excessive consumption of such yin foods did not take place at that time. Large webs between the fingers are becoming common among modern babies, and are often surgically removed after birth.

J.   Space between the fingers.   If the fingers are held closed and viewed from the back of the hand, and no space is showing, it is an indication of well-balanced nourishment. If spaces show between the fingers, it is caused by certain nutritional deficiencies, especially in the proportion among carbohydrates, proteins, fats and minerals, and reflects imbalances in the physical and mental constitution in general (Fig. 81). Accordingly, it has been said traditionally that if a person has a space between his fingers, he is unable to keep what he receives—a sign of misfortune.

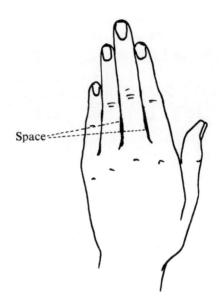

Fig. 81 Space between the Fingers

Space

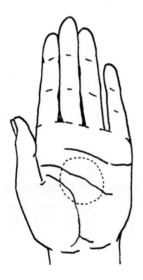

Fig. 82 Center of the Palm

K. Color of the center of the palm. The center of the palm is slightly indented (Fig. 82). If that region does not have a clean and clear color, and if it feels rigid and tight with slight pain when it is pressed, there is general physical and mental fatigue caused by underactive digestive and circulatory functions, resulting from an imbalanced diet. A change of color in this area reflects disorders arising in certain systems of the body, as follows:

Color	*Affected Systems*
Red	Circulatory
Purple	Respiratory and reproductive
Dark	Excretory
Yellow	Liver and gallbladder functions

This color change also arises on the base of the palm and wrist on the inside of the hand, and we can diagnose the corresponding conditions in the same way as for the center of the palm.

Fig. 83   Points at the Base of the Palm

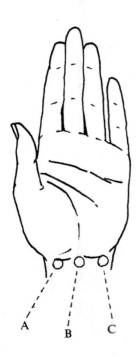

A   B   C

L.   Swollenness at the base of the palm.   If we press along the bony, fleshy region at the base of the palm, and swollenness arises at the wrist joint immediately under the palm, the following disorders can be diagnosed (see Fig. 83):

—Swollenness arising at point A, under the base of the thumb, indicates disorders in the lungs and respiratory functions, and the large intestine and its functions.

—Swollenness at point B, under the center of the hand, shows disorders in the circulatory and reproductive functions.

—Swollenness at point C, under the base of the little finger, shows disorders in the heart and circulatory functions, as well as in the small intestine and its functions.

M.   Curved fingers.   When the fingers are stretched, they should be straight and well-balanced in general. If certain fingers curve toward the inside or outside of the hand, it shows that certain organs and functions in the body tend to be overactive or underactive due to dietary imbalances during the periods of pregnancy and childhood growth (Fig. 84). As described later in *Oriental Psychodiagnosis*, these fingers correspond with certain functions in the body according to meridian flow. General correspondences are as follows:

Finger	*Corresponding Organs and Functions*
Thumb	The lungs and their functions
Index finger	The large intestine and its functions
Middle finger	The three chakras, and the circulatory functions
Ring finger	The three chakras, and the function of energy adjustment

Finger	Corresponding Organs and Functions
Little finger	The heart and small intestine and their functions

If the fingers curve toward the middle finger, it shows a disharmonious condition caused by the overconsumption of yang foods, including animal food, overcooked food, and oversalted food. It they curve away from the middle finger, the cause is the overconsumption of yin foods, including sugar and sweets, fruits and juices, raw vegetables—especially of tropical origin—beverages, alcohol, chemicals and drugs.

Fig. 84   Curving Fingers

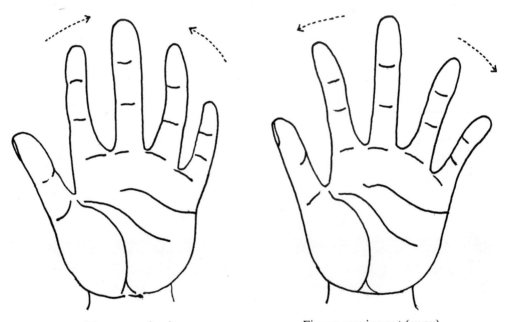

Fingers curving in   Fingers cuvring out (away)

N.   The length and height of the fingers.   If the fingers are stretched to full length, under normal balanced conditions the longest is the middle finger; second, the index finger; third, the ring finger; and fourth, the thumb and little finger. In height—their apparent length when viewed together on the hand—the highest should be the middle finger; next, the index and ring fingers; next, the little finger; and last, the thumb. The height of the ring finger should be between the level of the middle finger and the thumb.

However, different physical constitutions produce different lengths and heights. If the index finger appears taller than the ring finger, it shows a native weakness in the large intestines; and if the ring finger appears taller than the index finger, approaching the height of the middle finger, it indicates possible disorders in the heart, stomach or small intestines. If the little finger appears taller than the midpoint between the heights of the middle finger and the thumb, it shows that chronic disorders in the heart and small intestine may easily arise.

3. Shape of the fingertips

The tips of the fingers have different shapes, depending upon differences in constitution. General guidelines are as follows (Fig. 85):

Fig. 85   Forms of the Fingertips

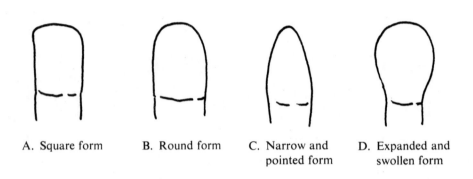

A. Square form   B. Round form   C. Narrow and pointed form   D. Expanded and swollen form

A. Square fingertips show that the parents were physically strong and hardworking people, and the mother consumed more yang animal food with less vegetable food during the pregnancy. This square fingertip shows a character that is physically active, determined, theoretical and aggressive.

B. Round fingertips show that the parents were healthy, and the mother ate mainly yang, well-cooked grains and vegetables, with less animal food, during pregnancy. They show a gay, active, energetic and positive personality, with understanding and sympathy.

C. Narrow, pointed fingertips show that the mother ate more yin, vegetable foods with less cooking, including fruits, sweets and other yin foods during pregnancy, and these were also eaten during the childhood growing period. They show a physical tendency to be more weak, and a mental tendency to be more sensitive and delicate, with an esthetic and artistic character, interested in the arts and metaphysical problems.

D. Expanded, swollen fingertips show the consumption of yang animal food with yin sugar, fruits, juices and sweets, resulting in an offensive, aggressive, self-centered and discriminating character. If the thumb has this shape, like the head of a poisonous snake, it shows that the father had a very wild, aggressive personality.

4. Special conditions of the fingertips

Since the fingertips are a point of discharge for excess energy, through the skin and the meridians, their condition often changes, showing changes in the internal condition of the body:

A. *Cracked, split fingertips* show that excess yin foods are being actively discharged, including sugar and sweets, fruits and juices, soft drinks and chemicals, drugs and medications. The internal functions are in disorder, including the circulatory, excretory and reproductive functions. Sexual weakness, impotence, and frigidity often appear in this condition.

B. *White, fatty skin* on the fingertips shows an accumulation of fat from both animal and vegetable sources, and especially and overconsumption of dairy products. The digestive and lymphatic systems are often disordered, and the kidneys and liver may be forming cysts or tumors. There may also be fat and mucus accumulating in the lungs.

C. *Red or purple fingertips* are caused by the overconsumption of yin foods. The lungs and respiratory functions, and heart and circulatory functions are abnormal. Over-sensitivity, nervousness, irritability, and depression are occurring, as well as changes of mind.

D. *Hard, flaky skin* on the fingertips shows the overconsumption of dairy products and other animal fats, along with excessive protein, mainly from animal sources. Hardening of the arteries and muscles is arising, along with rigidity in both body and mind. The overconsumption of eggs can also cause this condition.

E. *Soft, peeling skin* on the fingertips results from the overconsumption of liquid and sugar, including all beverages, fruits and juices, alcohol and other drinks, as well as drugs and medications. The heart and circulatory function, and the kidneys and excretory functions are now overactive. Mentally, oversensitivity and emotional irritability are present.

The Nails

As in the case of all peripheral parts of the body, the nails are a form of elimination of excessive nourishment, especially minerals, proteins and fats.

As long as eating continues, the growth of the nails also continues. The nails therefore show the physical and mental condition during the growing period, including the present condition. Guidelines for diagnosis are as follows:

1.   The color of the nails

Like the color of the lips, the color of the nails shows the quality of the blood. There are several types of color which change daily according to changes in the physical condition, due to changes in diet, activity, and other daily influences.

   A.   Pinkish red nails show a sound blood condition and generally healthy and balanced physical and mental conditions. If a person who has suffered from a chronic disease begins to show this color in his nails, caused by dietary improvements, it indicates that his condition is improving.

   B.   Reddish-purple nails show an abnormal blood condition caused by the overconsumption of yin foods, including dairy products, sugar and other sweets, fruits and juices, fats and oils, chemicals and drugs, as well as stimulant beverages. The digestive, circulatory and excretory functions are abnormal, with insomnia, constipation, diarrhea, fatigue, depression and many other physical and mental disorders.

   C.   Dark red nails show a higher content of fatty acids, cholesterol, and/ or minerals in the blood, due to the overconsumption of animal food, including meat, poultry, eggs, and dairy products, with salt. The heart and circulatory function, and the kidneys and excretory function are overloaded, and there is underactivity of the liver, gallbladder, and often the spleen. Hardening of the arteries and muscles, and inflexibility of the mind often occur.

   D.   Whitish nails indicate underactive blood circulation, and low hemoglobin—anemia in general. This condition is caused by dietary imbalance, including an overconsumption of refined flour, fruits, juices, sugar and other sweets. However, the overconsumption of salt, dried foods and animal foods, or a lack of liquid, may cause a similar condition, through constriction of the blood vessels and capillaries. The accumulation of fat and mucus in and around the heart, liver, pancreas, prostate and ovaries may be occurring. Leukemia and other forms of cancer often show this color in the nails. People in normal health do not have this whitish color in the nails, although it easily appears when the fingers are stretched, especially on the thumb and index fingers.

2. *The shape of the nails*

Variations in the shape of the nails are caused by dietary differences over many years, resulting in differences in constitution. General guidelines for diagnosis are as follow (Fig. 86):

Fig. 86   Forms of the Fingernails

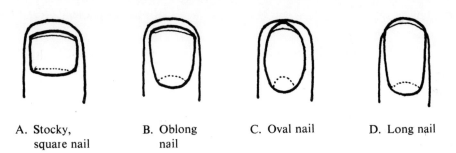

A. Stocky, square nail	B. Oblong nail	C. Oval nail	D. Long nail

A.   Stocky, square nails show a more yang constitution resulting from a diet of animal food, well-cooked grains and vegetables, with salt. There is a tendency to be physically active, but mentally inflexible.

B.   Oblong nails result from a diet of yang, well-cooked grains and vegetables with little salt and animal food. Salad, fruits and juices also contribute to a small extent. The constitution is more physcially and mentally balanced, but with some tendency toward rigidity.

C.   Oval nails are caused by more vegetable-quality foods, including lightly-cooked vegetables, with occasional fruits and juices. Eggs and dairy food may contribute somewhat. The constitution is physically weaker, but mentally more active with some emotional sensitivity.

D.   Long nails result from a diet tending toward less-cooked and raw vegetables, with fruits and juices, sugar and sweets, and other yin foods. The physical constitution is weak, especially the digestive and respiratory systems, and the mentality is oversensitive.

3. *Special conditions of the nails*

A.   Hardness and thickness.   Harder and thicker nails result from the overconsumption of food rich in protein and fat from both animal and vegetable sources, showing physical and mental strength and vitality. On the other hand, softer and thinner nails result from more vegetable-quality food,

Fig. 87   Various Conditions of the Nails

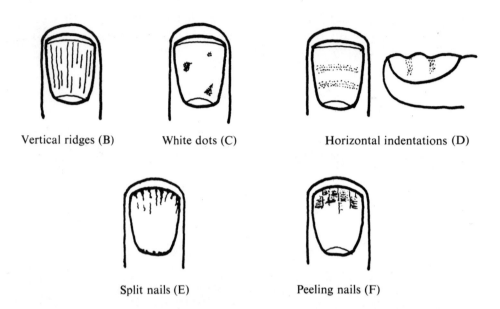

Vertical ridges (B)   White dots (C)   Horizontal indentations (D)

Split nails (E)   Peeling nails (F)

with stimulant beverages such as coffee and alcohol. Sugar and sweets as well as other yin foods and drinks also contribute. There is a tendency to be physically flexible and weak, but mentally active, with esthetic appreciation.

B.   Vertical ridges on the nails are the result of imbalanced nourishment —an overconsumption of carbohydrates and salt, and a lack of proper protein and fat. The digestive, liver and kidney functions may be underactive, and general fatigue appears.

C.   White dots on the nails show the elimination of sugars, including cane sugar, honey, syrups, fruit sugars, milk sugars, alcohol, chocolate, and any other sugars. The location of the spot on the nail shows the approximate date the sugars were eaten. Normally, an adult's nail grows in six to nine months. If the entire nail grew during a six-month period, and the white spot appears at the middle of the nail, the large amount of sugar was eaten three months ago. If the spot is located one-third of the way up the nail from the root, such sugar consumption occurred two months ago.

D.   Horizontal indentations in the nails show changes in diet. The person may have moved to a different climatic zone where his diet underwent a natural change, or if remaining in the same place, he made a significant change in dietary habits. For example, if a horizontal indentation appears one-third of the way from the tip of the nail, the dietary change took place four months ago, if the entire nail grows during six months. If another indentation is present one-third of the way from the bottom of the nail, such changes took place twice—two months ago and four months ago.

E.   *Split nails.*   If the ends of the nails are split or uneven, it indicates a chaotic dietary practice, and especially an overconsumption of yin foods and drinks. This condition shows that the circulatory, reproductive and nervous systems are in disorder, especially the functions of the testicles and ovaries, and that the nervous reactions are subnormal. If one thumbnail shows this condition, and the other thumbnail is normal, it shows that the testicles or ovaries corresponding to the abnormal side are malfunctioning.

F.   *Peeling nails.*   Peeling nails have the same cause as detachment of the retina, since the firmly attached layers of the nails have begun to detach. This condition is caused by the overconsumption of fruits, juices, soft drinks, vitamins, chemicals, drugs and medications, which deprive the body of minerals, producing a nutritional imbalance. Indigestion, gas formation, fatigue, menstrual irregularity, sexual weakness, depression, nervousness, insomnia and many other conditions are arising.

G.   *White moons* at the base of the nails differ according to personal condition. An active metabolism including activity in physical and mental growth and change shows white moons, while a slow metabolism shows smaller moons or no moons. Accordingly, during childhood and youth, everyone usually has moons, but this varies during adulthood, and the moons generally disappear during old age.

A physically active but less mentally active person tends to have larger moons, while a physically inactive but mentally active person tends to have smaller moons. However, very large moons show abnormal conditions such as oversensitivity and physical weakness due to the excessive consumption of yin foods and drinks.

7. The Feet

As one of the major peripheral parts of the body, the feet and toes, like the hands and fingers, represent the entire physical and mental constitution and condition, and correspond to various parts of the major organs and their functions. Specific conditions of the feet and toes reveal certain conditions of the organs, systems, and their functions, as well as the mental tendencies associated with these conditions.

The hands have a more expanded form, and correspond more to the upper and lower areas of the body including the lungs, heart, small intestines and large intestines. On the other hand, the feet, which have a more compacted form, represent more the organs located in the middle region of the body, including the liver and gallbladder, spleen, stomach, pancreas, kidneys and bladder. Furthermore, it can be said that the arms and hands represent the horizontal relationship between the central part of the body and the periphery, while the legs and feet represent the vertical relationship.

1. General characteristics of the feet

A. Size.   The size of the feet varies from person to person. The size of the feet, including both length and width, is generally proportional to the size of the entire body, but there are proportional differences due to individual constitution.

Larger feet indicate that the organs in the middle region of the body, such as the liver, gallbladder, spleen, pancreas, stomach, and kidneys are sound and active. Smaller feet show that the organs in the upper and lower parts of the body are more sound and active, including the lungs and large intestine, and the heart and small intestine. In general, those who have larger feet have more mental tendencies, including better intellectual and esthetic comprehension, while those who have smaller feet have better physical vitality and tolerance.

B. Height.   If the top of the foot is higher, it shows a more physically active nature, due to the consumption of comparatively more protein and minerals. If the top of the foot is lower and flatter, it shows a more mentally active nature, caused by the consumption of more carbohydrates and liquid. A person with a higher foot usually has a more narrow foot, while a person whose foot is lower usually has a wider foot.

C. The arches. Higher arches are due to more tightly contracted muscles, allowing more active functioning of the feet. This condition is caused by a comparatively low intake of liquid, fruits, juices and other yin foods. Lower arches are due to looser muscles and tissues, and show a tendency to be less physically active but more mentally active, especially in esthetic, artistic and religious comprehension. A higher consumption of the yin foods named above is indi-

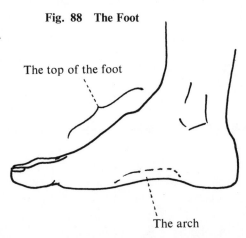

Fig. 88 The Foot

The top of the foot

The arch

cated. High arches are essential for athletes, sportsmen, dancers, and other physically active professionals, while lower arches are more common among thinkers, writers, muscians and artists, as well as religious persons.

D.   Joint flexibility.   The joints of the ankles and toes should be flexible and able to move freely in all directions. However, many modern people are losing this flexibility due to hardening of the arteries, muscles and joints, resulting from the overconsumption of foods high in cholesterol and saturated fats. Animal protein treated with salt also causes this inflexibility. Flexibility of the feet and toes shows not only physical lightness and mobility, but also mental adaptability. As this flexibility decreases, the entire lifestyle becomes more rigid and less adaptable to the constantly changing natural and social environment.

E.   Width of the foot.   If the width of the foot at the ball is narrower than normal—about one-third of the length of the foot or less—it is caused by the consumption of more yang foods, including food of both animal and vegetable types, with less liquid, and shows a more physically active and mentally sharp nature (Fig. 89).   If the width is more than one-third of the length of the foot, it is caused by more vegetable-quality food, and more yin foods, including salad, fruits and liquid. In this case, there is less physical activity and more esthetic and metaphysical comprehension.

Fig. 89   Width and Length of Foot

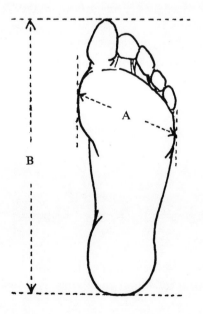

The proportion between the width (A) and and the length (B) of the foot is normally about 1:3.

Fig. 90   Protruding Ball of the Foot

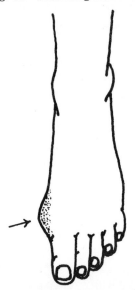

F.   Protruding ball of the foot.   Sometimes an abnormal, hard protrusion develops at the ball of the foot (Fig. 90). This may have begun to develop shortly after birth, or during adulthood. This protrusion has been called traditionally a "sign of a widow," or a "sign that he will become alone in old age." This condition shows hardness in the middle region of the body, in the area of the liver, stomach, pancreas or spleen, due to a one-sided diet: for example, carbohydrate and salt, protein and salt, fat and salt; or the overconsumption of salts or minerals. It indicates physical rigidity, especially in the middle region of the body, and mental rigidity with a tendency toward domination, discrimination, prejudice and jealousy. Although those who have this condition are more active in social life, these mental characteristics often lead to separation from family and friends.

G.   Feet that turn in or out.   If the feet turn outward while walking, it is due to constriction at the base of the spine, caused by the overconsumption of animal food, and shows a more aggressive, progressive and outgoing character both physically and mentally. In women, it may indicate a retroversion of the uterus. On the other hand, if the feet turn inward while walking, the area at the base of the spine is more open, due to the consumption of more vegetable-quality foods, and indicates a more gentle, conservative and introspective character, both physically and mentally.

Among western people, feet that turn outward are more common, while there are more people in oriental countries whose feet turn inward. Also, feet that turn outward have become more common in modern times, while feet turning inward are seen more often in the older generations. If they are in good health and following sound dietary practices, men should have feet that are straight or slightly turning outward, and women should have feet that are straight or slightly turning inward.

2.   The color of the feet

The feet should have the same clean, clear color as other parts of the body. Abnormal colors show certain disorders:

A.   Red.   A red color generally arises at a peripheral area of the foot— the toes, sides or back. It is due to the expansion of blood capillaries in these regions, caused mainly by the overconsumption of liquid and other yin foods, including sugar and sweets, fruits and juices, soft drinks and chemicals, drugs and medications. It shows that the heart and circulatory system are now overactive, with a faster pulse and rate of breathing, together with over-active kidney and excretory functions, often including frequent urination. Mentally, loss of clear thinking and general fatigue is indicated.

 B. Purple. A purplish color also appears at the peripheral regions of the foot, and is caused by the overconsumption of very yin foods, including sugar and sweets, fruits and juices, and possibly more chemicals, drugs and medications. All functions of the major organs are in disorder, especially the circulatory, excretory and reproductive functions.

 C. Other colors such as yellow, dark, green, and white may appear from time to time in rare cases, especially at the peripheral regions of the feet. They indicate that certain organs and their functions are abnormal. For example:

Color	*Condition and Cause*
Yellow	Liver and gallbladder disorders, due to the overconsumption of meat, poultry, eggs, and fats from both animal and vegetable sources.
Dark	Underactive kidney and excretory functions, due to the overconsumption of animal food, salt, baked flour products, well-cooked food, and other yang foods and drinks.
Green	Spleen and lymph functions as well as the blood circulation are abnormal due to the overconsumption of foods that produce fat and mucus, such as fatty meat, eggs, dairy food, sugar, white refined flour, and others. This color may indicate the formation of cysts, tumors and cancer.
White	The heart and circulatory functions, and the intestines and digestive functions are under-active due to constriction of the heart, blood vessels and capillaries. This is caused by the overconsumption of animal fat, salts, or other yang foods and drinks. General anemia or anemia in the intestinal region may also pro-duce this color.

3. *The toes*

The toes are formed by the meridians, and therefore each toe and the area immediately extending from it represents certain major organs and their functions (see Fig. 91).

Fig. 91   Areas of the Feet Correlating with Areas of the Body

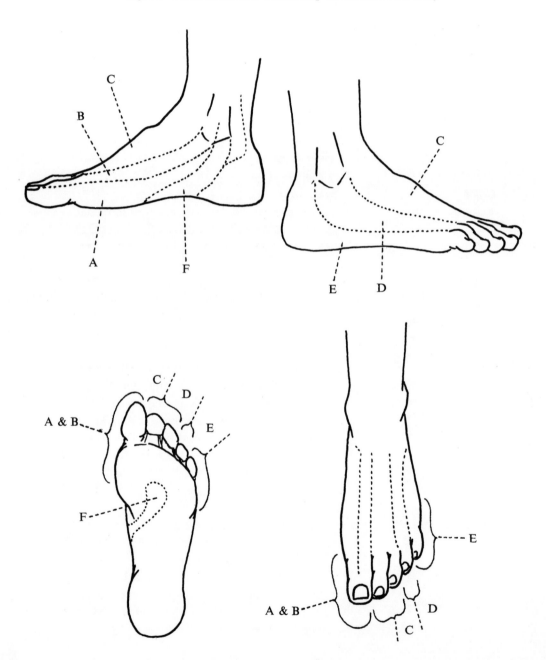

Toe and Extended Area	*Organs and Functions*
The first toe	The spleen, pancreas, and liver (A—Spleen and pancreas; B—Liver.)
The second and third toes	The stomach (C)
The fourth toe	The gallbladder (D)
The fifth toe	The bladder (E)
On the sole of the foot, the central part of the knuckle region	The kidneys (F)

These correlations also apply to the area immediately extending from each toe or point, as illustrated in Fig. 91. Accordingly, abnormal conditions appearing in certain toes and their connected areas show disorders in certain organ and their functions. For example:

Fig. 92   Callouses on the Feet

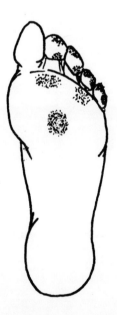

A.   *Hardness at the tips of the toes* is an indication that the corresponding organs and their functions are stagnated, possibly due to overeating and overdrinking, as well as a possible imbalance in the amounts of minerals, proteins, fats, carbohydrates, or vitamins concumed.

B.   *Callouses* show the elimination of excessive fat and mucus, caused by the overconsumption of food in general, or by imbalanced nourishment (Fig. 92). This elimination arises from a malfunctioning organ through its meridian. For example, if a callous appears on the fourth toe, the gallbladder and its functions are now abnormal due to the overconsumption of dairy products and other fats from both animal and vegetable sources. If a callous arises on the sole of the foot at the central part of the knuckle region, causing pain while walking, it shows an elimination from the kidneys through their meridian. In this case, there has been an overconsumption of foods such as flour products, fats and oils, and sugar and sweets, from both animal and vegetable sources.

   C. *Abnormal colors* appearing on certain toes or their extended areas show that the corresponding organs and functions are overactive, usually due to an overconsumption of yin foods and drinks (Fig. 93). If a green color appears on the inside of the foot toward the area below the anklebone, the spleen and lymphatic system may be developing a cancerous condition. Similarly, a green color appearing on the fifth toe and its extended area at the outside of the foot, below the outer anklebone, shows that a cancerous condition may be developing in the uterus, ovaries, or prostate. If a green color appears on the top of the foot in the extended area of the second and third toes, cancer may be developing in the stomach. And, the liver and gallbladder may be developing cancer if a green color appears on the fourth toe and its area extending from the fourth toe to the front of the foot below the anklebone.

Fig. 93   Examples of Color Change in Some Cases of Cancer

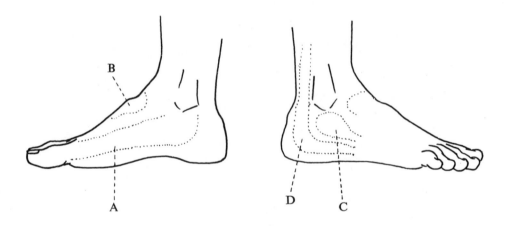

Light green coloration arises in the area corresponding to the location or kind of cancer:

    A.   Cancer in the spleen, pancreas, and lymph as well as Hodgkin's disease.
    B.   Cancer in the stomach area.
    C.   Cancer in the gallbladder area.
    D.   Cancer in the bladder, uterus, ovaries and prostate areas.

   D. *Two diagnosis points.*   Two points formed by the junctions of bones extending up from the toes can be used for diagnosis of the internal organs: (1) the indented point in the small valley formed by the junction of the bones extending up from the first and second toes; and (2) from the fourth and fifth toes (Fig. 94). If pain is felt when point (1) is pressed, it shows temporary disorders in the stomach and liver, due to overeating and overdrinking. General physical and mental fatigue are indicated as well. If pain is felt when point (2) is pressed, it shows that the gallbladder and bladder and their functions are in disorder, due to the overconsumption of food and drink, and especially of salt and fat. There is a tendency toward general fatigue and sleepiness. It may also indicate contraction of the gallbladder, and the formation of cysts or stones in the gallbladder.

Fig. 94   Two Diagnosis Points on the Foot

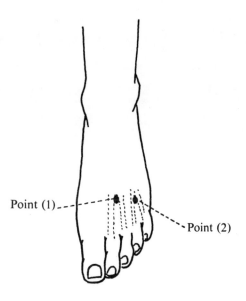

Point (1)

Point (2)

Fig. 95   Length of the Toes

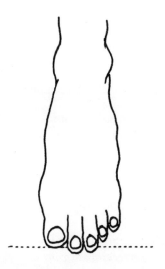

Second and third toes longer than the first toe shows weakness of the stomach.

E.   Length of the toes.   From the first toe to the fifth toe, the length of the toes gradually decreases. However, in many people, the second and/or third toes are longer than the first toe (Fig. 95). This is caused by dietary habits during the embryonic period that have caused weakness in the stomach and its functions. In this case, there are possible stomach disorders including gastritis, ulcers, cancer and other diseases.

F.   Curving toes.   If the first toe curves abnormally toward the second toe, it shows that the spleen and lymphatic functions are overactive, while the liver functions are underactive, due to the consumption of excessive fats and oils from both animal and vegetable sources, and

Fig. 96   Curving Toes

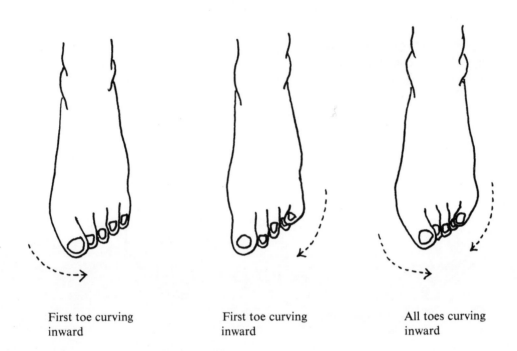

First toe curving
inward

First toe curving
inward

All toes curving
inward

more yin foods and drinks in general. If the fifth toe curves abnormally
toward the fourth toe, it indicates overactivity in the kidneys, bladder, and
their excretory functions, caused by the overconsumption of yin foods and
drinks, including all beverages, fruits, juices, sugar and sweets.

G.   *The toenails.*   Under normal conditions, the toenails should be harder
than the fingernails. The condition of the toenails, including their color,
varies according to the individual condition:

1.   *The normal color of the toenails* is pink, and slightly darker than the
     fingernails. The surface of the toenails should be smooth, showing
     balanced nourishment and healthy activity.
2.   *Darker colors in the toenails* including dark blue and dark purple
     show imbalanced nourishment, due to the overconsumption of yang
     animal food, or yin foods such as fruits and sugar, or both.
3.   *White color and rugged surfaces* often appear on the toenails, espe-
     cially the fourth and fifth nails. This condition is caused by the over-
     consumption of liquid and sometimes fat, including all beverages,
     fruit, fruit juice, dairy products, and fats and oils from both animal
     and vegetable sources. Disorders in the liver and gallbladder as well
     as the kidneys and excretory system are indicated.

4. *The soles of the feet*

The soles of the feet correspond to the entire body, and each area of the sole corresponds to a certain part of the body. Such physiotherapies as foot massage, reflexology and moxibustion use this correlation in order to release stagnation from various organs and systems. Fig. 97 shows the correlation between the bottom of the foot and certain related areas of the body.

Fig. 97   Areas of the Sole of the Foot Corresponding to Areas of the Body

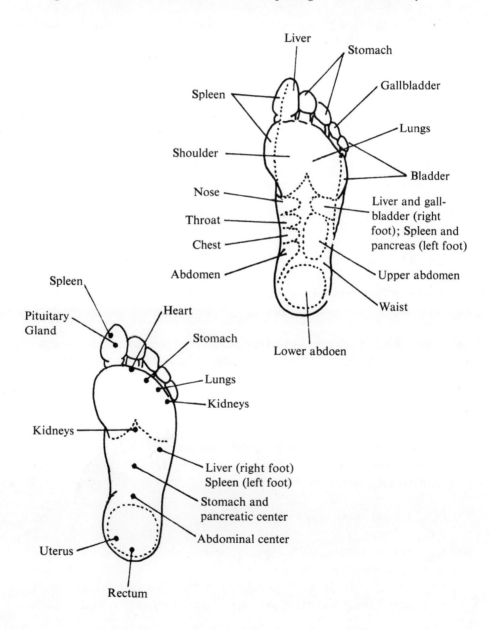

When certain areas of the sole show hardening, tension, and pain when they are pressed, it shows that the corresponding organs and functions are in disorder. These disorders are mainly caused by the stagnation of energy flow and blood circulation due to overconsumption of animal foods, foods rich in fat from both animal and vegetable sources, sugar and fruits, as well as liquid.

If the sole of the foot is soft and elastic when pressed, it shows that the metabolism of the physical and mental conditions is harmonious. If symptoms of hardness and pain increase, it shows that physical and mental disorders are developing more toward degeneration. These internal disorders can often be alleviated through the application of proper therapeutic treatment together with correction of the diet.

5. Peeling skin and athlete's foot

Athlete's food is often accompanied by a condition of peeling skin on and between the toes, as well as the rupture of skin between certain toes, making walking difficult. Although athlete's food often shows germ activities in the area, the real cause is the overconsumption of liquid, including all beverages, fruits, fruit juices, sugars and sweets, and some chemicals and drugs, as well as other yin types of food. These foods produce a condition of heavy humidity in the region of the toes, leading to ruptures and encouraging germ activities.

8. Skin Diagnosis

As the periphery of the body, the skin reflects its antagonistic and complemental partner, the inner depths of the body. When the internal organs and glands become disordered, symptoms always appear on the skin. The condition of body fluids such as the blood and lymph also appears on the skin. Because the main function of the skin is adjustment between the external environment and internal body conditions, it also reflects environmental change. Diagnosis of the condition of the skin generally focuses on three major characteristics: (1) the condition of the skin, (2) the color of the skin, and (3) marks appearing on the skin.

1. The condition of the skin

Normal, healthy skin should be clear, smooth, slightly shining, and slightly moist. If other conditions are present, it is the result of disorders arising in some part of the body. As all physical and mental disorders are due to disorderly dietary habits, abnormal skin conditions are also caused mainly by dietary habits. In the modern arts of beauty care, external treatments are emphasized more than internal change through diet, and endless efforts are made with unsatisfactory results. However, a beautiful skin develops naturally as a result of a balanced macrobiotic diet.

A.   *Wet skin.*   This condition is easily detected if the palm is unusually wet. The palm as well as all other surfaces of the body should maintain a condition of slight moisture, but not of wetness. The cause of this condition is the overconsumption of liquid, including watery cooking, beverages, fruits, juices, milk, and all other fluids. Sugar and other sweets also produce water within our body.

Wet skin indicates thinner blood, rapid metabolism, faster pulse, and excessive perspiration and urination. This condition produces various physical and mental disorders, including epilepsy, vertigo, diarrhea, fatigue, dull thinking, forgetfulness, detachment of the retina, glaucoma, hair loss, and pains and aches in various parts of the body such as the ears, teeth and gums.

The water balance in our body is reflected in the number of urinations per day, which should normally be three or four, in the case of adults. Some medical advice which recommends a large liquid intake is not advisable in many cases except as a temporary measure to recover from dehydration, to eliminate poisons or excessive animal foods from the body. The desire for water is proportional to the volume of salts, protein and carbohydrates consumed, and therefore the comprehensive approach of dietary change is required for a long-term alteration in liquid intake.

B.   *Oily skin.*   Normal skin is slightly oily, but if an excessively oily condition is present—often on the peripheral parts of the body such as the forehead, nose, cheeks, hair or palms—it is caused either by the overconsumption of oils and fats, or by disorders in fat metabolism. This condition shows that the liver, gallbladder and pancreas are not functioning normally. The lungs and respiratory functions, and the kidneys and excretory functions are also affected.

Often, oily skin also reveals certain related symptoms such as the formation of stones in the gallbladder and kidneys; the formation of cysts and tumors in the breasts, ovaries, uterus, and other parts of the body; pancreatic disorders, including diabetes; mucus accumulation in various parts of the body; hearing difficulties, cataracts, sclerosis; and many others.

The intake of all fatty foods including meat, poultry, eggs, animal foods, sugar, flour products, fruits and juices, and vegetable oils should be minimized in order to relieve this condition. The overconsumption of protein and carbohydrates can also cause oily skin, and therefore, less eating is advisable.

C.   *Dry skin.*   Dry skin is caused either by dehydration or by the overconsumption of fats and oils. The first cause is more common among moderm people. Medical personnel generally advise increased oil consumption to relieve a dry skin condition, but this is rather ineffective: a dry skin surface is often caused by the formation of fat layers under the skin, which prevent the elimination of moisture toward the surface. Therefore, the diet should be adjusted toward the elimination of fats and oils.

Dry skin shows that there is a relatively large amount of fat and cholesterol in the bloodstream. The accumulation of fat and cholesterol around the heart and in the arteries, as well as in major organs such as the liver and gallbladder, lungs and intestines, spleen and pancreas, and the prostate and uterus, is common in this case. There may also be hardening of the arteries, irregular pulse, mental rigidity, and the formation of cysts, tumors and cancer in some cases. There is probably abnormal tension near the affected organs and along the related meridians. In order to heal this condition, it is adviseable to eliminate all meat, poultry, eggs and dairy products, as well as sugar and sweets from the diet.

D. Rough skin. This condition has two possible causes: (1) overconsumption of protein and heavy fats, or (2) overconsumption of sugar and sweets, fruits and juices, soft drinks, drugs and chemicals. A condition with the first cause is more difficult to change. The second condition is characterized by more open sweat glands and, usually, a slightly red color.

Rough skin of the first type reflects an internal condition that includes hardening of the arteries, and accumulation of fat and cholesterol around the organs and in the arteries. Usually, the liver and kidneys are affected. The accompanying symptoms often include the appearance of protein in the urine, intestinal disorders, muscular tension, pains and aches in the joints, stiffness of the neck and shoulders, general fatigue and mental rigidity.

In the second case, rough skin indicates disorders of the circulatory, excretory and nervous functions. Symptoms often include irregular pulse, excessive sweating, frequent urination, diarrhea, vertigo, excessive sensitivity, and emotional instability.

In both cases, rough skin can be corrected by reducing the intake of animal food, fats and oils, sugar and sweets, fruits and juices, and drugs and chemicals, and by the practice of balanced dietary habits.

E. Doughey skin. This skin condition is common among modern people. The skin appears whitish and flabby, and lacking in active elasticity. It may appear anywhere on the body, but usually more on the front, including the face, chest and abdominal regions. The cause is mainly the overconsumption of dairy products, sugar, and refined flour products.

Doughey skin indicates that fat and mucus are accumulating in various parts of the body such as inside the forehead, in the nasal cavities, inner ear, breast, lungs, liver, gallbladder, kidneys, uterus, ovaries, prostate, and the thyroid glands. Accompanying symptoms often include hay fever, hearing difficulties, coughing, spitting mucus, the formation of cysts and tumors in the breast, uterus, ovaries and prostate regions, tightness of the arteries, vaginal discharge, formation of stones in the kidneys and gallbladder, general fatigue, cloudy thinking and laziness. There is also the potential for the development of cancer.

The consumption of more grains and vegetables can correct this condition, along with the elimination of animal fats, dairy products, sugar, and refined flour products, and the reduction of fruits, juices, beverages and oils in the diet.

2. *The color of the skin*

The color of the skin is different in every person. There are commonly-known differences in skin color among persons of different racial backgrounds: white for Caucasians, darker for Latins, yellow for Orientals, coppery for Middle Easterners, brown for East Indians and Central and South Americans, dark or black for Africans, and blue-black for native Australians. However, these differences in skin color are not primarily racial, since skin colors are the result of the influence of the external environment and the internal condition and nourishment. The principles of skin color can be summarized as follows:

—A colder and cloudy climate produces whiter skin, and a warmer and sunnier climate produces darker skin.
—More yang foods produce lighter skin, and more yin foods produce darker skin.

For example, the Negro race, living in Africa, develops a dark or black color due to the warm climate and to the consumption of tapioca, bananas and other yin tropical products, while their color tends to change if they move to North America and consume more yang animal products as well as dairy foods. Among the yellow races, it is well known that the skin color tends to change toward white if they move to a more snowy region and consume saltier foods which are cooked for a longer time.

Aside from these natural skin colors, there are many abnormal colors that may appear because of disorders in the physical condition. These colors appear not only on the surface of the skin, but also in any part of the body, including the hair, eyes, lips, and nails as specified in the other chapters of this book. The most common abnormal colors appearing on the surface of the skin can be summarized as follows:

Color	Cause	Conditions
Red	Excessive yin foods and drinks, including liquid, fruits, alcohol, sugar, sweet, spices, and stimulants.	Expansion of capillaries. Heart and circulatory disorders. Lung and respiratory disorders. Nervous disorders. Emotional instability.
Yellow	Excessive yang foods and drinks, including meat, eggs, fish, seafood, salt and minerals, and vegetables such as carrots, pumpkin and squash.	Disorders of the bile functions of the liver and gallbladder. Pancreatic disorders. Kidney and excretory disorders. Emotional aggressiveness.
Purple	Extremely yin foods and drinks, including fruits and juices, sugar and sweets, drugs, medications, and chemicals.	Intestinal and digestive disorders. Nervous disorders. Sexual and hormonal disorders. Fear and despair.
White	Excessive yang animal food rich in fat, including all dairy products, or the overconsumption of salts and minerals.	Contraction of blood capillaries and tissues. Nervous alertness. Liver, gallbladder, kidney, and especially spleen and lymph disorders. Stubborn and narrow mind.
Blue	Excessive yang animal food and salts, with yin sugar and sweets, alcohol and stimulants. Food rich in carbohydrates.	Malfunction of the liver. Disorders of the spleen and pancreas functions. Anger and short temper.
Brown	Excessive yang animal food and yin vegetables, both rich in protein and fat. Sugar and sweets, fruits and juices.	Intestinal and digestive disorders. Kidney and excretory disorders. Discrimination and prejudice.
Dark	Excess yin food, including sugar and sweets, fruits and juices, drugs and	Kidney and excretory disorders, intestinal and digestive disorders, sexual

Color	Cause	Conditions
	chemicals.	and hormonal disorders. Depression and fear.
Green	Excessive yang food rich in protein and fat, or excessive yin food rich in sugar and oils. Chemicals, drugs and medications.	Decompsition of tissues or cells. Development of cysts, tumors and cancer. Emotional insecurity and arrogance.

3. Marks on the skin

Many marks appear on the skin throughout life. At birth, there are usually no marks on the skin, although there are some exceptions. A newborn infant may have a green patch at the bottom of the buttocks, known among Asian societies as the "Mongol's Mark;" or there may be vivid red or brown patches on certain parts of the body, as when the mother has taken drugs or medications during pregnancy. The so-called "birth mark" is such a case. For similar reasons, a newborn baby may have black spots known as "beauty marks" as evidence that the mother experienced a disease or high fever during

Fig. 98   Examples of Beauty Marks along the Lung Meridian

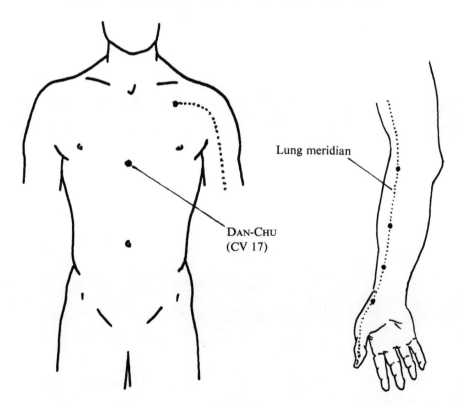

Lung meridian

DAN-CHU
(CV 17)

her pregnancy, though it is comparatively rare.

Most marks appearing on the skin arise after birth, since they are symptoms of the elimination of certain excesses caused by dietary imbalances or adjustments by sickness. These marks include the following:

A. Black spots. Known as "beauty marks," these appear in the vicinity of acupuncture points along the meridians through which internal and external energy comes into or goes out of the body. They also appear at the junction of connecting tissues.

These black spots show the elimination of carbon compounds produced by the burning of excess carbohydrates, proteins and fats within the body. Accordingly, they appear after a disease accompanied by a high fever, such as pneumonia, bronchitis, stomach and intestinal fever, and kidney and bladder infections. By observing the location of these spots, and especially the meridian along which they are located, it is possible to determine in which organ the disease was experienced. For example, black spots appearing along the lung meridian show that pneumonia or bronchitis occurred in the past. The same kind of spots appearing in the chest region, especially at the point DAN-CHU (CV 17), show that a past disease involved infection of the heart region.

Therefore, black spots appearing on the face can indicate weakness in certain systems, organs or glands, and the resulting physical and mental tendencies. In this way, by observing the black spots, we can also understand personal character. Fig. 99 provides some common examples.

Fig. 99   Some Examples of Facial Beauty Marks

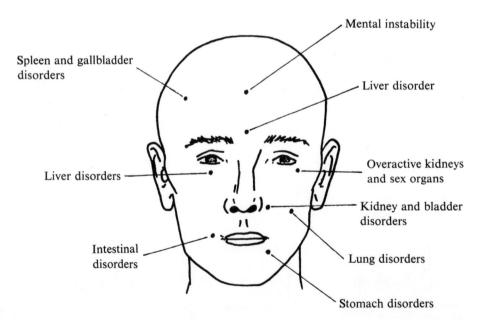

Mental instability

Spleen and gallbladder disorders

Liver disorder

Liver disorders

Overactive kidneys and sex organs

Kidney and bladder disorders

Intestinal disorders

Lung disorders

Stomach disorders

B.   *Dark brown patches*, *or freckles*, appear often in modern people. They occur on the more peripheral and exposed parts of the body such as the face, hands, arms, and shoulders, as well as here and there throughout the body. The tendency of freckles to appear more in the upper part of the body is due to their cause.

Freckles are the elimination of excessive carbohydrates, especially mono- and disaccharides, including refined sugar, honey, fruit sugar and milk sugar. The yin character of these substances is more attracted to yang sunlight, and therefore, freckles are more likely to appear during the summer. A few generations ago they were called "death marks," especially when they appeared in a large size on the back of the hand. People who live in cloudy, darker climates, or who do not eat these sugars, do not have so many freckles. The elimination of these foods from the diet can cause a gradual disappearance of freckles.

If freckles appear more on certain meridians, or on the surface area corresponding to certain internal organs, we can say that the overconsumption of sugars has affected these related organs. For example, freckles appearing on the back of the hand and arm along the large intestine meridian show that the intestinal functions are somewhat in disorder due to sugar consumption. Similarly, freckles appearing on the shoulders indicate disorders in the intestinal functions.

C.   *Large brown patches* are known as MO-SHOKU (蒙色) in oriental medical terminology. Though their color is similar to that of freckles, MO-SHOKU are larger than freckles, and their appearance is more infrequent and temporary. They can appear on any part of the body corresponding to a disordered organ. Fig. 100 shows some examples.

If the MO-SHOKU disappears due to external treatment such as repeated moxibustion, it shows that the disorders of the corresponding organs have also disappeared, and normal functions have been recovered.

D.   *Moles*, which are tiny dark brown mounds, appear among some people. They are the elimination of excessive protein. This protein does not necessarily come from the consumption of protein itself, but is also produced by overeating in general, and especially overeating of carbohydrates and fats. For this reason, in the ancient Orient moles were known as a sign of an egocentric nature. Moles can naturally dry up and disappear, therefore, if the dietary habits are properly corrected.

Moles may appear (1) along the meridians, and (2) along the muscles. In the first case, the functions of the organs for which that meridian supplies energy have been affected by the overconsumption of protein or food in general. In the second case, the organ which correlates to that area of muscle has been affected by the same cause. The following are examples:

Fig. 100   Examples of Mo-Shoku

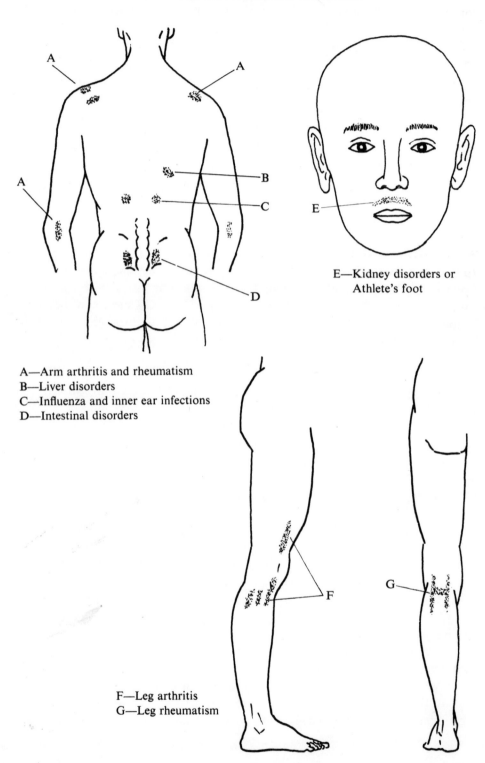

E—Kidney disorders or
Athlete's foot

A—Arm arthritis and rheumatism
B—Liver disorders
C—Influenza and inner ear infections
D—Intestinal disorders

F—Leg arthritis
G—Leg rheumatism

E. Warts may be skin color, or brownish and slightly darker than skin color. They are softer than moles, with an irregular shape. Warts are the elimination of a mixture of protein and fat, again caused by the overconsumption of these food elements or by overeating in general. However, warts tend to appear more in people who consume a large volume of fats or sugar. They can be eliminated by correction of the dietary habits. Warts also appear more on the upper part of the body, due to their slightly yin nature.

Warts can appear irregularly with no apparent relationship to the location of meridians and points, like freckles. They indicate general disorders in the digestive, circulatory and excretory functions. The organs especially involved are the large intestine, which is usually stagnated in this case; and the kidneys, which are usually accumulating fats. People who have warts have a tendency to develop cysts, tumors, and cancer in the breasts, colon and reproductive organs, as well as skin diseases, indigestion and urinary infections.

F. Pimples appear more on the upper body surface, because of their yin nature, caused by excessive fats, sugar and flour products. They are usually red and white, because of the expansion of blood capillaries and fatty tissues. Pimples usually appear on the cheeks, forehead, nose, the area around the mouth, jaws, shoulders, chest, and the back of the body more than in other places. The location of the pimples indicates that the corresponding organs are affected by the accumulation of fat and mucus. For example:

Location of Pimples	*Affected Organ or Areas of Body*
Forehead	Intestinal area
Cheeks	Lung area
Nose	Heart area
Around the mouth	Reproductive area
Jaws	Kidney area
Shoulders	Digestive tract
Chest	Lung and heart areas
Back	Lung area

Pimples can be eliminated by avoiding foods that directly contribute to the accumulation of protein and fat, mucus and excessive liquid in these organs and systems.

G. White patches appear often among modern people, and sometimes gradually spread over the body. These patches are caused by a constant intake of excessive dairy products, especially milk and cream. This condition indicates that the accumulation of fat and mucus has spread throughout the respiratory and reproductive systems. A hormonal imbalance often results, including thyroid, pancreatic and gonad functions.

This condition naturally contributes to the formation of cysts, tumors and eventually cancer, especially in the breast, colon, and reproductive areas.

A long time is required for gradual recovery of this condition, through the elimination of dairy products and the increase in consumption of grains and vegetables. However, if vegetable oils are used in excess, they can also cause a retardation of the healing process.

H. *Bluish patches*, which sometimes appear on the surface of muscle areas, are caused by stagnation in the bloodstream. This condition often arises during internal hemmorhage, due to broken capillaries caused by an external shock or by an internal expansion of the capillaries. However, if a balanced diet is being eaten, it is very rare that an external shock will produce these blue patches. Accordingly, the real cause of this condition is the overconsumption of yin foods: excessive fruits, juices, sweets, drugs and chemicals.

This condition indicates that the circulatory and urinary functions are not sound. Accompanying symptoms often include irregular pulse, frequent urination, emotional disturbance and nervousness. This condition can be gradually corrected by the recovery of sound blood quality with increased minerals.

I. *Varicose veins* appear mostly on the back and inside areas of the legs. They appear as expanded veins with a light green, light blue, dark red, or in some cases, dark purple color. They often appear in women at the time of pregnancy.

This condition shows disorders in the intestinal digestion and the excretory functions. It is also often accompanied by disorders in the liver, gallbladder, spleen or pancreas. Migraine headaches and irregular reproductive functions may be present as well.

Varicose veins are caused by excessive liquid, including all beverages and juices, as well as fruits. Excessive oil intake can also contribute. It is possible to improve varicose veins gradually by reducing the intake of these foods and beverages, and decreasing animal foods and salt, along with hot applications which accelerate the circulation of blood.

J. *Eczema*—dry, hard, raised areas of skin which may be white, yellow or reddish in color—often appears among modern people. It shows a massive elimination of excessive fats, mainly caused by the intake of animal foods, especially dairy products. Among dairy foods, cheese is the most notable contributor to this condition, and eggs cooked with butter can also contribute greatly.

This condition shows disorders in the circulatory and excretory functions, with an accumulation of fat and cholesterol in major organs such as the heart, liver and kidneys. There may be frequent cysts and tumors, and a tendency to develop cancer. Other symptoms include hardening of the arteries, dandruff, dry skin, insomnia, and emotional insecurity.

Eczema can be corrected by the elimination of all fatty food, with an increase in the consumption of grains, vegetables and seaweed.

All abnormal skin conditions, including those described above, are manifestations of the relationship between the internal environment within the body and the external environment. If the diet which nourishes the internal environment is properly adjusted according to the changes in the external environment—the seasons, the climate, the weather—in connection with daily physical and mental activity, a skin condition can be maintained which is a natural result of a sound internal condition.

Afterword

To know things is to know the self.
More knowing is a path to make us
    more humble and modest.
He who makes himself the lowest
Knows everything,
And he attains universal consciousness
Of eternal life.

This book has introduced the major ways of diagnosis based upon the principles of oriental medicine, in accordance with the understanding of the
order of the universe—the law of nature which constantly governs all phenomena throughout the universe, including our present life on Earth as
human beings. These methods of diagnosis have been developed and used
for the past 30 years through the observation of hundreds of thousands of
people, without analysis of the internal condition of the body, but only
through sharp observation reflecting from the pure state of nothingness. As
the present human race consists of four billion people upon this planet,
there are billions of variations in lifestyles and activities; and each one of the
billions of people has numerous changes and fluctuations according to natural
and environmental conditions, social and cultural influences, traditional and
ancestral contributions, and personal variations in eating and activity. As a
result, the scientific study of diagnosis—without the use of any analytical,
divisional modern methods which often have harmful effects upon our health,
as in the use of X-rays, radiation, blood analysis, bone-scan tests and many
other applications—needs unlimited depth of understanding of humanity
and its relation with the order of the universe. It requires many years of
observation and examination, and reflection upon the surrounding conditions. This is the study of humanity itself.

To master this practice, to develop penetrating insight into the various
physical and mental disorders and their underlying causes, requires well-
being, especially a clear mind and a clean body. The master of diagnosis has
a profound understanding of nature and of humanity. His judgement can
work instantaneously and intuitively in direct apprehension of the totality
of the object he is seeing, as if he himself is the universe which produces
these patients, affirms their existence, changes their conditions. In other words,
the master of diagnosis lives with universal consciousness, without any
tendency toward discrimination, prejudice or narrowness, and with infinite
compassion and patience.

The contents of this book are merely an introduction of the guidelines
of some of the major methods of diagnosis, presented in the hope that everyone can easily understand antagonistic and complemental relations as a

balancing factor in all phenomena—that is yin and yang. In the early stages of learning how to diagnose, the application of antagonistic and complemental relationships is very practical and useful. However, a more advanced practice of diagnosis is done intuitively and almost unconsciously, beyond the scope of any theory, logic or mechanical techniques. In order to acquire such ability, it is essential for the student of diagnosis to continuously observe balanced macrobiotic dietary practices, including whole cereal grains, vegetables, beans and seaweed as a major part of the daily diet. He or she should extend love and help to all other people, inspiring them toward a healthier life, guiding them toward a happier life.

Needless to say, the practice of diagnosis is not limited to those methods which have been introduced in this book. This art has many more dimensions, some of which are almost impossible to describe in writing, but which require demonstration and direct explanation with examples. In this category is *vibrational and spiritual diagnosis*, which has the following general purposes and methods of practice:

1.   This kind of diagnosis involves the perception of vibrations that are usually invisible and which arise along with our physical and mental functions. By examining them through observation, direct experience, and the use of the senses—seeing, hearing, smelling, tasting and touching—we can distinguish disorders that may be developing in the depths of the internal organs.

2.   In this way, we can examine all major thought processes including memories, visions, tendencies of thinking, attachments and detachments, delusions, illusions and future visions, in order to diagnose physical and mental conditions.

3.   With this kind of diagnosis, we can also study the quality of the aura, or vibrations discharged from inside the body, together with environmental forces and dietary energy, understanding environmental conditions and dietary practices.

4.   This diagnosis furthermore reveals the influences of the so-called spirits or ghosts of dead persons, or living persons at a distance, and the disorders caused by these spiritual influences. By clarifying their cause, we can suggest how to purify these spiritual influences and secure physical and mental well-being.

5.   Through this kind of diagnosis, we can see the influences of ancestral heredity which have developed from generation to generation—generally for the past seven generations, and eventually up to a few thousand years ago. By revealing these ancestral influences in the physical and mental constitution, it becomes possible to foresee a person's future as well as the destiny of his offspring.

6.   Furthermore, this kind of diagnosis develops a direct understanding, intuitive but practical, of a person's reincarnation: of his previous lives—not

only of the immediately past life, but of many past lives—and his future reincarnations—again, not only of the next life but of several lives in the future.

7.   Through this way of diagnosis, we can further examine not only someone's condition, but also the conditions of his family, relatives and friends with whom he has had some sort of relations; and the nature of the society and community within which he is presently living, within which he lived during his past lives, and within which he will live during his future lives.

The immediate purpose of diagnosis is to assist people in the improvement of their health and the realization of their well-being. However, the ultimate purpose of diagnosis is to understand the endless process of the development of life, which is changing forever, covering the entire dimension of this infinite universe—in other words, the understanding of the infinite scale of life with the most deep, high and unlimited consciousness. Therefore, if diagnosis is approached only in a mechanical way, without a constant effort to develop universal consciousness and a high personality with compassion, it is nothing but the same witchcraft into which the modern techniques of diagnosis have degenerated.

As the author of this book, I wish to urge all readers to use the arts of diagnosis and the information presented in this book not only as techniques, but also as a means to understand the human race, including the reader himself, for the development of higher consciousness. This book of diagnosis was not written to give its readers knowledge and techniques, but to prepare an open gate into the new era of humanity, through the recovery of our various disorders; and to establish eventually one healthy and peaceful world of mankind.

Although the contents of this book are introductory, I sincerely hope this information will not be used to criticize or devaluate other people, and that the readers who use these arts of diagnosis will maintain a spirit of modesty and gratitude to all people, surroundings, nature and the universe, and its infinite order. I wish to have all readers use this book as a guide for helping each other, and as a guide for reflecting upon our own constitutions and conditions, in order to realize the endless happiness of humankind.

> MICHIO KUSHI
> Brookline, Massachusetts
> Christmas Day,
> December 25, 1979

Index